DAILEY'S NOTES ON BLOOD
Second Edition

John F. Dailey

Medical Consulting Group
25 Atherton St.
Somerville, MA 02143
1-800-851-8518

Published by
Medical Consulting Group
Somerville, MA

Layout by
Desktop Support Consultants
Medford, MA

Artwork: Jordan P. Dailey
Cover Design: Susan Keller

ISBN: 0-9631819-2-0
Printed in the United States of America
97 96 95 94 93   10 9 8 7 6 5 4 3 2

CONTENTS

CHAPTERS

FIGURES

CHARTS

PREFACE

The tissue blood is responsible for the total physiology of human beings. It is a fascinating topic, but also a highly complex one. Because standard texts on hematology cannot be understood without a knowledge of chemistry, the author wrote this book, *Dailey's Notes on Blood*. It is a comprehensive guide to blood – and the reader does not have to know chemistry to readily achieve an understanding of the basics of blood, its function, origins, components, and disorders.

Dailey's Notes on Blood is designed for ease of use. Information is presented in concise form, with important vocabulary terms in the margins. Illustrations depict important concepts of blood. Each chapter has self-check questions. At the back of the book are answers to questions, a glossary, and an appendix of charts showing normal blood values.

Medical Consulting Group, the publisher of this book, offers technical training programs and publications pertaining to blood and related topics for companies and healthcare professionals.

Medical Consulting Group
25 Atherton Street
Somerville, MA   02143
800-851-8518
fax: 617-623-3319

ABOUT THE AUTHOR

John F. Dailey has two decades of experience in various aspects of blood – both in surgery and in industry. Dailey was involved in multiple trauma treatment, operations of the heart bypass pump and other types of equipment while working with surgeons at Emerson Hospital in Concord, Mass.; St. Elizabeth's Hospital in Brighton, Mass.; and Maine Medical Center in Portland, Maine.

Dailey worked in industry for medical equipment manufacturers training physicians and allied health personnel on the use of autologous blood recovery systems in the surgical setting. He also conducted clinical trials on new products; for example, one that collects and processes wound drainage blood and another that is revolutionizing the treatment of ischemic heart disease.

Dailey has a B.A. in Biology, St. Francis College, has done graduate studies in biochemistry and physiology at the University of Rhode Island and Brandeis University, and has specialized training in Cardiovascular Perfusion at Northeastern University.

1 AN INTRODUCTION TO THE CONCEPT OF BLOOD

What Is Blood?

Hematology is the study of blood and blood-forming tissues. It includes blood's function, diseases, use in treatment such as in surgery, and role in conditions such as anemia and leukemia. Hematology is primarily concerned with the formed elements, or cells, of the blood system: red cells (erythrocytes), white cells (leukocytes), and platelets (thrombocytes), all of which are suspended in the liquid medium of blood: plasma.

Blood can be thought of as a transportation system, with the arteries, veins, and capillaries functioning as the roadways. As blood circulates throughout the body it transports oxygen from the lungs to the tissues of the body, where it is released in the capillaries to the various tissues. Digestive products absorbed in the intestine are distributed to the various tissues by the blood. Waste products from the tissues are picked up by the blood plasma and excreted (eliminated) from the body through the skin, lungs, and kidneys.

The formed elements have different functions. The white cells in blood are involved in the body's defense against microorganisms and foreign material. Red cells are involved in the transport of oxygen and carbon dioxide throughout the body. Platelets are essential in preventing blood loss (hemostasis).

The volume of blood present in the circulatory system (arteries, veins, capillaries) is called the total blood volume. The average adult has four to eight liters (1 liter = 1000 mls, or 1.06 qts.) of blood. Cellular elements comprise 45% of the blood volume, and plasma comprises 55%. Plasma is a viscous (sticky) fluid that is 90% water and 10% solid matter, the latter being comprised of carbohydrates, proteins, lipids, salts, vitamins, and enzymes. Whole blood refers to formed elements and plasma, i.e., blood as a whole.

hematology

plasma

white cells
red cells

platelets

total blood
volume

whole blood

1

Figure 1 STEM CELL PRODUCTION IN BONE MARROW,
OR HEMATOPOIESIS

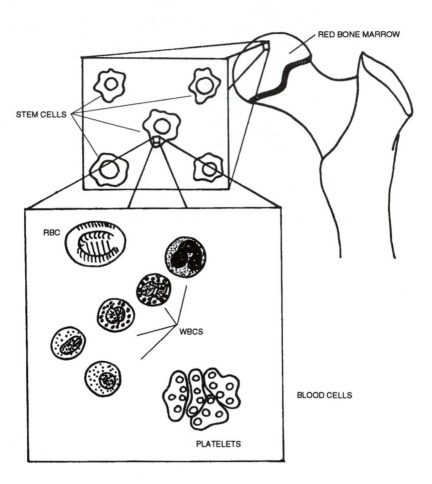

The Origin of Blood

Hematopoiesis is the term used to describe the production of blood cells. (See Figure 1.) During early fetal development hematopoiesis takes place in the liver, spleen, and thymus. After birth and continuing on into adulthood most blood cell production occurs in the bone marrow. (See Figure 2.)

hematopoiesis

There are two types of bone marrow found in the body: red and yellow. Both types consist of a spongy, fibrous matrix and are found in the center of bones. Yellow marrow is not involved in blood cell production and is 96% fat. Red marrow, which is the hematopoietic marrow, is 75% water and 25% solid matter (proteins, carbohydrates, salts, etc.). In young children, red marrow can be found in the cranium, ribs, pelvis, sternum, and vertebrae.

hematopoietic (red) marrow

The Blood Cells

Each kind of cell (red, white, and platelet), or formed element, has its own function. (A cell is referred to as a formed element.) Blood cells differ structurally from each other, and each cell has its own characteristic life span. The number of cells in the blood at any time is constant, because the production and destruction of the cells are balanced.

formed element

Figure 2 BLOOD CELL DEVELOPMENT

 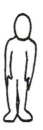 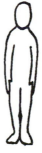

FETUS

LIVER,
SPLEEN,
THYMUS

CHILD

BONE MARROW OF
SKULL, RIBS, STERNUM,
VERTEBRAE, PELVIS

ADULT

BONE MARROW OF LONG BONES
OF ARMS AND LEGS, RIBS,
VERTEBRAE, STERNUM

3

Figure 3 BLOOD CELL DIFFERENTIATION

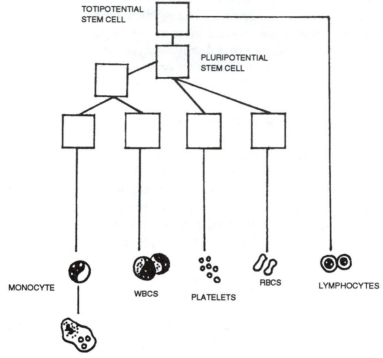

Figure 4 STEM CELL DIFFERENTIATION

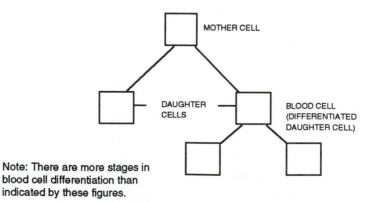

Note: There are more stages in
blood cell differentiation than
indicated by these figures.

Just as human beings go through the various stages of the life cycle — from birth to death — so do blood cells. In order for them to carry out their intended functions blood cells must be fully mature. In a healthy person only mature blood cells are found in the circulation, but in persons with disease states, immature and abnormal cells may be present.

The stem cells (totipotential and pluripotential) in the red marrow produce different kinds of cells. Granulocytes, erythrocytes, thrombocytes, and monocytes originate from a common stem cell, the pluripotential stem cell. The totipotential stem cell gives rise to both lymphocytes and the pluripotential stem cell. (See Figure 3.)

stem cells

The stem cells have two major functions: 1) the replication or generation of more stem cells and 2) the generation of differentiated daughter cells. The differentiated "daughter cells" eventually become blood cells.

differentiated daughter cells

When a stem cell divides it forms two "daughter" cells. Both are identical to the original stem cell, which is called the mother cell. One of the daughter cells remains a stem (or committed) cell so that the generating process can continue as the need for more blood cells arises. If both stem cells were to become blood cells, there would be no pool of stem cells to divide and thus no blood cells to replace the ones in circulation. The other daughter cell matures and becomes a blood cell, either a red cell, white cell, or platelet. (See Figure 4.)

mother cell

THE CONCEPT OF BLOOD / QUESTIONS

1. What are the formed elements of blood? The liquid medium in which they are suspended?

2. Explain how blood can be compared to a transportation system.

3. What is a function of platelets?

4. Describe plasma and its components.

5. What does the term hematopoiesis mean and where does it occur in the adult?

6. Describe two characteristics of blood cells.

7. Name the two kinds of stem cells.

8. Describe the role of the differentiated daughter cells in the production of blood.

2 THE CIRCULATORY SYSTEM

The circulatory system is a closed loop (continuous) system of the body providing channels through which blood travels as it delivers nutrients and oxygen to organs and tissues of the body. (See Figures 5, 6, and 7.) Other terms used to describe this system are the vascular space or vascular system. Blood or fluid within the vascular system, or space, is said to be intravascular, and when outside the vascular system, extravascular. (See Figure 8.)

vascular space/
vascular system
intravascular
extravascular

Fluid continually circulates between the blood and tissues. This fluid consists of proteins, nutrients, hormones, metabolites (waste products of metabolism), and electrolytes that maintain equilibrium between the blood and tissues of the body. Fluid and plasma components that leave the vascular system enter the interstitial space where they then become available to enter the tissue cells. Interstitial space refers to the space surrounding the cells outside the vascular system.

interstitial
space

The channels of the vascular system are the arteries, arterioles, capillaries, venules, veins, and indirectly the lymphatic system. (See p. 11.) Arteries are thick-walled muscular vessels used to carry blood away *from* the heart. Veins are thinner walled, do not contain the musculature that arteries do, and carry blood *to* the heart. (See p. 12.) Arterioles, or smaller arteries, become progressively smaller and eventually become a mass referred to as a capillary bed or capillary network. Once inside the organs and tissues the small arterioles become capillaries, the smallest vessels of the vascular system. Capillaries are one cell layer thick. Capillary beds are throughout organs and tissues. The channels of the vascular system are lined with flat cells called endothelium.

arteries

veins

capillary bed

capillaries

endothelium

The major artery leaving the heart is the aorta, which has many branches of smaller arteries arising from it to supply blood to various organs and tissues. As the arteries approach the organs and tissues they decrease in

aorta

Figure 5 CIRCULATORY SYSTEM

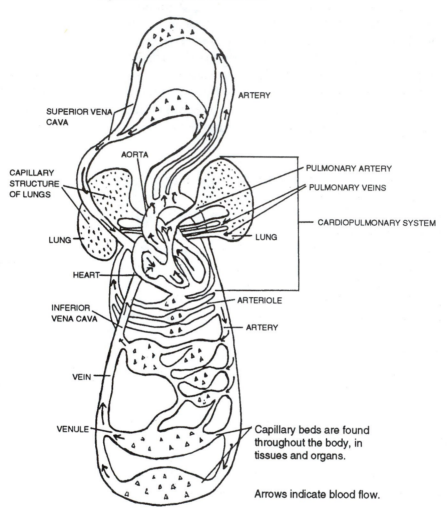

ARTERY

SUPERIOR VENA CAVA

AORTA

CAPILLARY STRUCTURE OF LUNGS

PULMONARY ARTERY

PULMONARY VEINS

CARDIOPULMONARY SYSTEM

LUNG

LUNG

HEART

ARTERIOLE

INFERIOR VENA CAVA

ARTERY

VEIN

VENULE

Capillary beds are found throughout the body, in tissues and organs.

Arrows indicate blood flow.

Figure 6 DETAILED STRUCTURE OF A CAPILLARY NETWORK

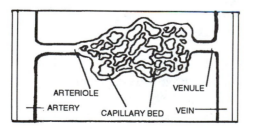

ARTERIOLE

VENULE

ARTERY

CAPILLARY BED

VEIN

size and become what is known as arterioles. Once inside the organs and tissues, small arterioles become capillaries.

arterioles

Capillaries are the smallest vessels of the vascular system. They are 1 millimeter (mm) long and 7-9 microns (μ) in diameter and penetrate and abound in every organ and tissue of the body. The capillary network is referred to as the microvasculature. It is at the capillary level that an exchange of nutrients, gases, hormones, waste products, etc. takes place between blood and tissues. The capillaries have pores in their endothelial lining that expand and allow substances to pass between the blood and tissues by a process of diffusion. Once proteins and other large molecular weight substances pass through the capillary pores and leave the vascular system, they often cannot return through the pores and are then picked up by a network of vessels called the lymphatic system, which returns them to the circulation. The fluid that does not leave the vascular system in the capillary bed is returned through venules to the veins and on to the heart.

microvasculature

Figure 7 VASCULAR SYSTEM

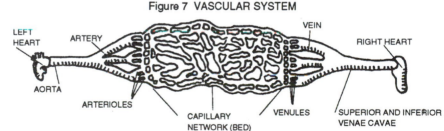

LEFT HEART · ARTERY · VEIN · RIGHT HEART · AORTA · ARTERIOLES · CAPILLARY NETWORK (BED) · VENULES · SUPERIOR AND INFERIOR VENAE CAVAE

Figure 8 BLOOD-TISSUE INTERFACE

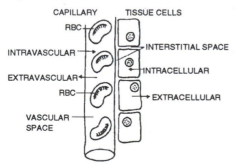

CAPILLARY · TISSUE CELLS · RBC · INTERSTITIAL SPACE · INTRAVASCULAR · INTRACELLULAR · EXTRAVASCULAR · RBC · EXTRACELLULAR · VASCULAR SPACE

9

Figure 9 LYMPHATIC SYSTEM

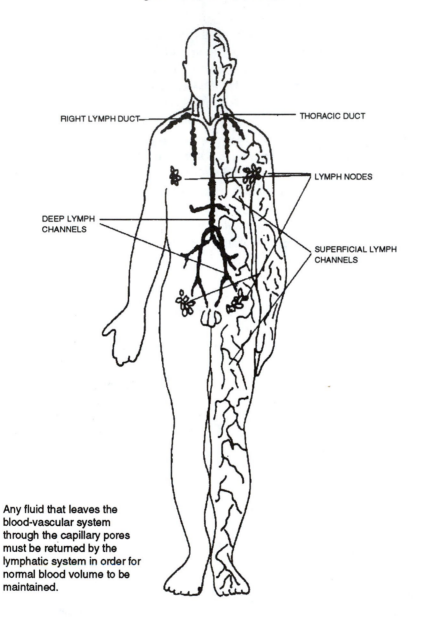

RIGHT LYMPH DUCT

THORACIC DUCT

LYMPH NODES

DEEP LYMPH CHANNELS

SUPERFICIAL LYMPH CHANNELS

Any fluid that leaves the blood-vascular system through the capillary pores must be returned by the lymphatic system in order for normal blood volume to be maintained.

The Lymphatic System

The lymphatic system is a network of capillary-like vessels, ducts, nodes, and organs that help maintain the fluid environment of the body. Like the blood-vascular system, the lymphatic system is made up of a system of channels. It does the following: 1) picks up fluids and large complex substances that have left the circulatory system and entered the tissues and 2) returns them to the vascular system via the thoracic and right lymphatic ducts.

The lymphatic system does not form a closed loop system as does the vascular system. Lymphatic vessels begin as tiny, unconnected capillary-like structures in tissues. These structures merge to form progressively larger vessels that are interrupted at various sites by small filtering stations called lymph nodes.

lymph nodes

Eventually, lymphatic vessels drain into two large lymph vessels, the thoracic duct, on the left side of the body, and the right lymphatic duct, on the right side. (See Figure 9.) These two vessels empty into veins in the upper chest and return fluid to the vascular system.

thoracic duct
right lymphatic duct

Fluids leave the vascular system to maintain equilibrium within the vasculature and to provide nutrients to the cells outside it, i.e., in the interstitial space. If fluid remains in the interstitial space, the person develops a balloon-like appearance. Blood volume is quickly depleted, meaning fluid is lost from the circulation.

Fluids of the body require constant circulation, and the pump that maintains this circulation is the heart. The heart propels fluids through the blood-vascular system. Any fluid that leaves this system through the capillary pores must ultimately be returned to the vascular system by the lymphatic system in order for normal blood volume to be maintained.

11

The Peripheral Circulation

The vascular system includes both the peripheral and cardiopulmonary systems. The peripheral circulation refers to the circulatory system, but not to the cardio-pulmonary (heart and lungs) circulation.

arteries
aorta
arterioles
capillaries

venules

Think of the circulatory system as one large continuous loop. Arteries take blood from the heart and veins return blood to the heart. They branch from the aorta and become smaller to form arterioles, which branch further to form capillaries. At the distal (farthest) end of the capillaries, the smallest veins form. These are called venules. As venules return blood to the heart, they become progressively larger. The veins return blood to the heart via the two major veins of the body, the superior vena cava and the inferior vena cava. The superior vena cava receives venous blood from the head and upper part of the body, whereas the inferior vena cava receives venous blood from the lower part of the body. These two vessels enter the right atrium of the heart. (See Figure 10.)

Figure 10 HEART

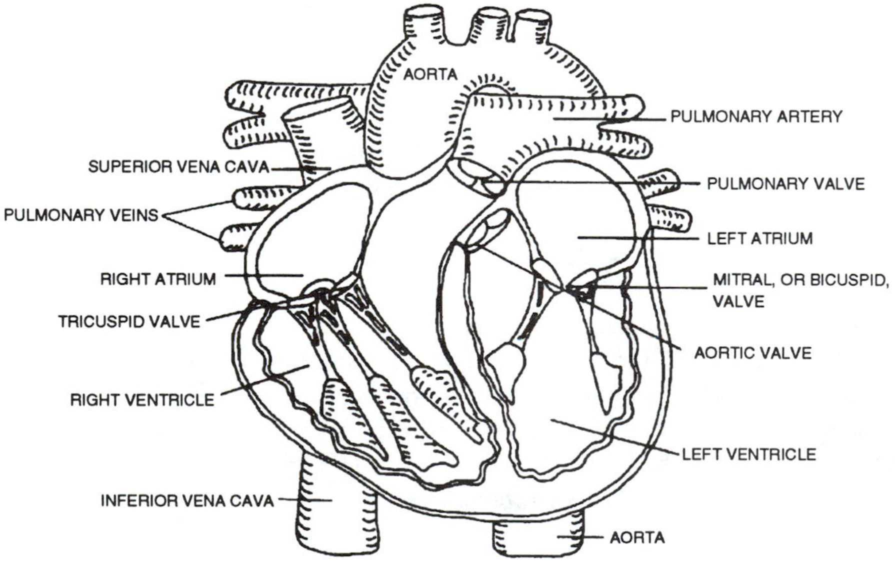

AORTA
PULMONARY ARTERY
SUPERIOR VENA CAVA
PULMONARY VALVE
PULMONARY VEINS
LEFT ATRIUM
RIGHT ATRIUM
MITRAL, OR BICUSPID, VALVE
TRICUSPID VALVE
AORTIC VALVE
RIGHT VENTRICLE
LEFT VENTRICLE
INFERIOR VENA CAVA
AORTA

12

The Cardiopulmonary System

The cardiopulmonary system refers to the heart and lungs as they function together. (See Figure 11.) The heart pumps blood throughout the body and to the lungs where blood receives oxygen. Deoxygenated blood (blood low in oxygen and high in carbon dioxide) returns from the organs and tissues of the body via the inferior and superior venae cavae to the right atrium (RA) of the heart. Blood in the right atrium is pumped to the right ventricle (RV) through the tricuspid valve. From the right ventricle deoxygenated blood is pumped out through the pulmonary valve to the pulmonary arteries to go into the lungs.

superior and inferior venae cavae
RA
RV

The lungs are large spongy organs filled with capillaries and alveoli. The microvasculature (capillary network) of the lungs is very large. In fact, if this system were removed and spread out it would be the size of a tennis court. The capillaries of the lungs form a close network with the alveoli, which are tiny air sacs within the lungs filled with oxygen. It is in the alveolar

alveoli

Figure 11 CARDIOPULMONARY SYSTEM

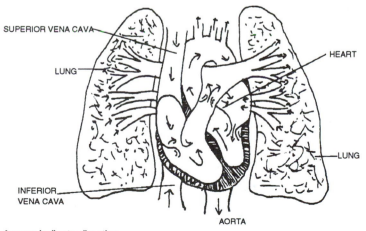

Arrows indicate direction of blood flow.

13

LA
LV

capillary network that oxygen (O_2) and carbon dioxide (CO_2) are exchanged. (Carbon dioxide is the waste product of cellular metabolism.) Once the exchange has taken place, blood is then oxygenated and returned from the lungs by the pulmonary veins to the left atrium (LA) of the heart. Blood in the left atrium is pumped into the left ventricle (LV) through the mitral, or bicuspid, valve. The oxygen-rich blood is ejected from the left ventricle through the aortic valve to the aorta. (See Figure 10.) From there, blood is distributed throughout the body via arteries, arterioles, and capillaries.

THE CIRCULATORY SYSTEM / QUESTIONS

1. Briefly explain the basic relationship between blood and the circulatory system.

2. What is another term for the circulatory system?

3. Name the channels of the vascular system.

4. Describe the path blood follows when it leaves the heart and goes to the tissues and organs.

5. What important function takes place at the capillary level?

6. What event takes place when large molecular weight substances leave the vascular system and cannot return?

7. What is the major function of the lymphatic system?

8. Why do fluids leave the vascular system?

9. What are the filtering stations of the lymphatic system?

10. What two vascular systems are included in the circulatory system?

11. The aorta, arteries, arterioles, and capillaries are the channels that take blood away from the heart to the organs and tissues. What channels return blood to the heart?

12. What is the lining of the vascular system called?

13. What is deoxygenated blood?

14. Describe the pathway of deoxygenated blood in the cardiopulmonary system.

15. What two gases are exchanged in the alveolar capillary network of the lungs?

16. Describe the course of oxygenated blood in the cardiopulmonary system.

3 THE IMMUNE SYSTEM

It has been only within the last few years that great strides have been made in understanding the immune system and how it functions. To have a working knowledge of blood one must also understand the immune system and its relationship to white blood cells, also called leukocytes. Basically, the immune system protects the body from microorganisms and foreign substances by attacking them and rendering them harmless. A complicated task faces the specialized organs, tissues, and white blood cells that make up the immune system: to recognize and destroy harmful invaders without causing damage to the body's own tissue. The process is known as phagocytosis and involves a number of the white blood cells: granulocytes, macrophages, T cells, and B cells.

phagocytosis

The immune system is unlike any of the body's other systems. It is not a system of channels like the circulatory system or an electrical network like the nervous system. In fact, the various components of the immune system do not stay put, but instead move freely throughout the body penetrating both fluids and tissues.

The best way to understand the immune system is to think of it as a highly trained and disciplined military unit. Like the military it consists of training and support groups, specialized units, and a highly skilled communications network. Surveillance units are constantly on the lookout for foreign invaders and provide the first line of defense for the body. When encountering foreign organisms they send out signals that activate other members of the unit to mount the necessary defense to prevent the invaders from reaching their target.

Microorganisms such as bacteria, viruses, parasites, and other invaders are called antigens. Actually, antigens are proteins on the surface of the invaders that the body recognizes as foreign. They are introduced into

antigens

the body by various routes, through the skin, mouth, blood, etc. The body recognizes antigens as foreign, or not part of "self." Technically, antigens are any group of microorganisms or foreign material that invades the body and causes the body to produce antibodies in response.

Antibodies, or Immunoglobulins

An antibody is a chemical complex produced by specialized B cells/plasma cells in response to a specific antigen. When the body recognizes an antigen a corresponding antibody binds with it to form what is called an antigen-antibody complex. (See Figure 12.) This complex is what is known as the immune response. The immune response causes other white blood cells to become activated in seeking out the complex and engulfing it.

antigen-antibody complex, or immune response

Antibodies, or immunoglobulins, are chemically complex protein molecules. They are produced by plasma cells in response to interactions among T cells, macrophages, and B cells. The B cell matures and becomes a plasma cell that produces an antibody in response to a particular antigen.

B cell
▼
plasma cell
▼
antibody

Figure 12 ANTIGEN-ANTIBODY COMPLEX

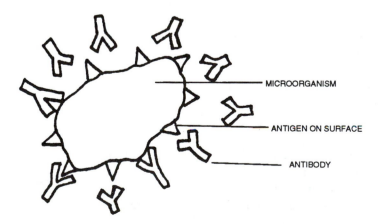

MICROORGANISM

ANTIGEN ON SURFACE

ANTIBODY

Immunoglobulins are divided into five classes and are released in a specific sequence within the immune response:

I. The first antibody produced on exposure to an antigen is IgM (immunoglobulin M). This is a large chemically complex molecule, that because of its size, is restricted within the vasculature; it cannot escape into the tissues. Its main function is to stimulate the complement system. (See p. 22.)

II. The second antibody produced in response to an antigen is IgD, about which little is known. Researchers believe this antibody assists the B cell in reacting to T cell stimulation causing the B cell to mature to a plasma cell that produces an antibody.

III. The third antibody is IgE, the antibody that is produced in excess in people who have allergies. Most of the white blood cells that rush to an attacked tissue's defense do so via the bloodstream. As white cells invade the area under attack the blood vessels dilate. In the process, the pores in the vessel walls stretch to a size sufficient enough for antigen-seeking cells to leave the blood and enter the tissues. IgE is specifically designed to release histamine, a chemical that causes pores in the vessel wall to dilate and allow white cells through. As soon as this occurs, IgE has performed its function.

IV. IgG, the immunoglobulin most important to humans, is also known as gamma globulin. It is divided into four subgroups, each of which has a specific purpose. IgG_1 protects the body from bacteria, but not from those organisms encased in a saccharide (sugar) coat; for example, meningococcus, pneumococcus, and gonococcus. To counter the saccharide-coated organisms, nature provides humans with IgG_2, to attack and destroy them. IgG_3 neutralizes certain types of viruses. Once inside the cell, however, such viruses are protected from the effects of antibodies, because antibodies cannot penetrate a cell's membrane. IgG_4

immunoglobulins

IgM

IgD

IgE

IgG
gamma globulin

19

is similar to IgE in that it produces potent vasodilators (substances that cause vessel pores to open). IgG_4 primarily provides protection for the bronchioles (airways) of the respiratory tract (lungs).

IgA

V. IgA, the fifth and final class of antibodies, protects mucus membranes (that line mouth, bladder, gut, nose, and vagina) and forms a protective barrier for these areas. IgA simply binds the antigen and immobilizes it so that the antigen-antibody complex can be removed with mucin, a viscous fluid produced by mucus membranes.

Cell-Mediated and Humoral Responses

The immune response is divided into two categories: cell-mediated and humoral. 1) Cell-mediated responses occur between antigens and specialized lymphocytes known as T cells. When the T cell recognizes an antigen it directs the B cell to produce antibodies specifically for that antigen. To produce the antibody the B cell turns into a plasma cell. When the antibody combines with the antigen on the target cell, the antigen becomes more palatable to the macrophages. Phagocytosis takes place when macrophages and granulocytes engulf the target cell. (See Lymphocytes, p. 49.) Cell-mediated responses happen before humoral responses. 2) Humoral responses are carried out by B cells/plasma cells through the production and circulation of antibodies in response to an antigen. For antibody production to take place, B cells must be stimulated by T cells. The activities of the T, B, and phagocytic cells conclude antigen destruction. Both cell-mediated and humoral responses are necessary for antibody production to occur.

Phagocytosis is the process by which white blood cells engulf material and render it harmless, usually through the action of enzymes located inside the phagocytic cells. It occurs in both humoral and cell-mediated responses. Phagocytosis will not occur unless stimu-

Figure 13 ANTIBODY PRODUCTION

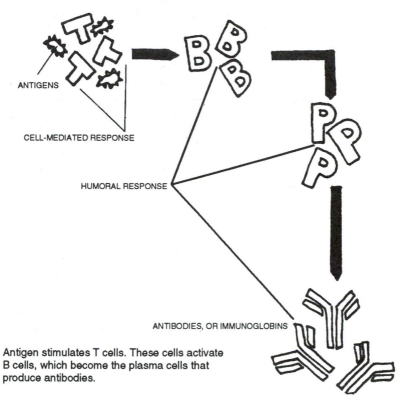

ANTIGENS

CELL-MEDIATED RESPONSE

HUMORAL RESPONSE

ANTIBODIES, OR IMMUNOGLOBINS

Antigen stimulates T cells. These cells activate
B cells, which become the plasma cells that
produce antibodies.

lated to do so. It depends on all the responses of the
immune system. Phagocytosis includes: T cell stimulation of the B cell/plasma cell; the coating of the target
cell antigens with antibody; and the adhesion of the
target cell with the macrophage, which allows the
macrophage to engulf the target cell. (See Figure 13.)

phagocytosis

Cell-mediated responses are crucial for combating
infections caused by microorganisms that reside and
multiply within cells. These include viral infections
and infections caused by bacteria that prefer intracellular attack (attacking the cell from the inside, rather
than outside the cell membrane). It is within the cell
that viruses replicate and do most of their damage.

21

The Complement System

The complement system works in conjunction with the immune system by defending the body from infections and foreign matter. The complement system involves over 18 distinct plasma proteins that react in sequence and bring about a number of biologically significant events. It is thought to provide a first-line defense before an immunological response (antibody production and cell stimulation) can be mounted. It also assists the macrophage, a large white blood cell, to adhere to cells coated with antibody or to cells coated with complement protein.

macrophage

When the complement system is activated in response to an infection or foreign matter, the patient benefits. It takes about a week before antibodies reach full force, and until then the complement system provides immune protection. The complement system helps defend the patient from infection by organisms that antibodies may not attack. It provides a line of defense against organisms that are not susceptible to antibodies and may actually go to work before the antibodies have time to kick in.

Both cell-mediated and humoral responses may sometimes be enhanced by other activities of the immune system, such as the complement system. When the body needs to remove foreign matter from itself, a phagocytic cell, such as a macrophage, is first stimulated to stick to the foreign matter and then to engulf it. Some bacteria and other organisms have surface antigens that bind (attach) immunoglobulins, thus causing the macrophage to stick to them. Other foreign substances, however, have capsules (outer coverings) that reduce the binding capability of immunoglobulins. If the immunoglobulin cannot attach itself to a foreign substance, the macrophage is repelled and phagocytosis does not occur. In this instance the complement system becomes activated and assists the macrophage in sticking to the surface of the foreign matter.

The complement system involves two distinct pathways (series of events): 1) the classical and 2) the alternative. Each pathway is stimulated to assist the immune system in different ways. (See Figure 14.) The classical pathway is usually activated when either IgM or IgG binds to antigens on the surface of microorganisms, thus enabling the macrophage to engulf the microorganism.

classical and
alternative pathways

The alternative pathway is activated by bacteria with polysaccharides (complex sugars) present on their surface membranes. Polysaccharides prevent antibodies from adhering to the bacteria and thus prevent macrophages from sticking to the bacteria and engulfing them. The alternative pathway provides complement protein that adheres to these bacteria and allows the macrophages to do the job of sticking to the bacteria and engulfing them.

Figure 14 COMPLEMENT SYSTEM

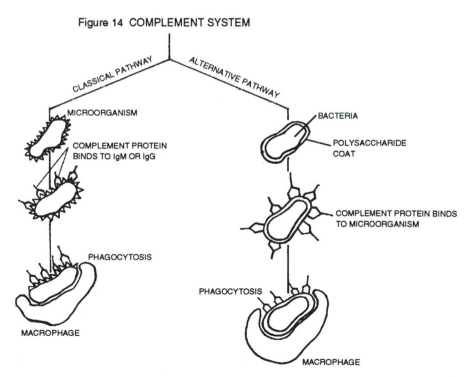

23

There are instances when the complement system becomes activated in the absence of organisms — during hemodialysis, open heart surgery, and when shed blood is collected intraoperatively and postoperatively. For reasons not really clear, foreign surfaces have the capability of stimulating the complement system. In the above instances, the complement system may be activated when hemodialysis tubing, or tubing used in open heart surgery, or the plastic container for shed blood is used.

hemolysis

The manifestations of complement system activation are usually directed against the red blood cell and cause hemolysis (destruction of the red cell membrane). Hemolysis is a potentially lethal situation for the patient. If it becomes widespread and a large number of red blood cells are destroyed, very few cells are left to carry oxygen to the tissues. Remnants of the red blood cell (stroma) may also then block the microvasculature of the lungs and kidneys.

THE IMMUNE SYSTEM / QUESTIONS

1. What is the primary function of the immune system?

2. Which blood cells are involved in the immune system? Provide two name designations.

3. Name three white blood cells.

4. Describe the process of phagocytosis.

5. Explain the term antigen.

6. What does the body do in response to the invasion of antigens?

7. What is an antibody? How is an antigen-antibody complex formed?

8. What is another term for the antigen-antibody complex?

9. What is another term for antibodies?

10. Describe how an antibody is produced.

11. Antibodies are produced by the body in a sequence within the immune response. Give one fact about each class of immunoglobins.

12. What is another term for IgG?

13. True or false. Antibodies cannot penetrate a cell's membrane.

14. Why are viruses protected from the effects of antibodies?

15. What are the two categories of the immune response?

16. Name the white blood cells that play a role in phagocytosis.

4 THE ABO BLOOD TYPING SYSTEM

Blood groups, or types, were discovered at the beginning of the twentieth century by Landsteiner, an Austrian hematologist. (See Figure 15, p. 28.) Blood types in the ABO system are determined by the presence of two distinct antigens (proteins) found on the red blood cell membrane. These antigens are inherited from the parents and are designated "A" and "B." Red blood cells with A antigen on their surface membrane are termed Type A, those with B antigen Type B, those with both antigens A and B Type AB, and those with neither antigen present Type O.

antigens A and B on cell membrane

Landsteiner also discovered two natural antibodies in the blood plasma: anti-A antibody and anti-B antibody. Anti-A antibody in Type B blood agglutinates (clumps) the cells in Type A blood. Anti-B antibody agglutinates Type B blood cells. Neither antibody agglutinates Type O blood cells, because they have no antigens on their membranes. Blood types are incompatible if the antigens on the red cell of the donor combine, or clump, with the anti-antibodies in the plasma of the recepient. Clumping occurs when blood types are incompatible. It occurs when the wrong blood type is used in transfusion and in a test to determine blood type. (See Figure 15.)

antibodies in plasma

Persons with Type A blood have anti-B antibody in their plasma; those with Type B blood have the anti-A antibody. The plasma of Type AB blood has neither antibody in it, whereas Type O blood has both anti-A and anti-B antibody in the plasma.

Medical personnel must be certain of the patient's blood type; it can be fatal if the wrong blood type is administered. When homologous (someone else's) blood is used it must be type specific to the patient. An A Type patient must receive Type A or O blood, a Type B patient Type B or O blood. A Type AB patient can receive the following: Type A, Type B, Type AB, or Type O blood. Type O can receive only Type O.

Figure 15 ABO BLOOD TYPING AND COMPATIBILITY

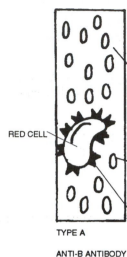 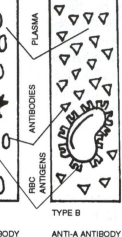 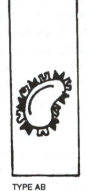 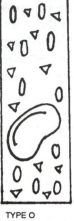

RED CELL

PLASMA

ANTIBODIES

RBC ANTIGENS

TYPE A

ANTI-B ANTIBODY

TYPE B

ANTI-A ANTIBODY

TYPE AB

NO ANTIBODIES
BOTH ANTIGENS

TYPE O

ANTI-A AND
ANTI-B ANTIBODY
BOTH ANTIBODIES
NO ANTIGENS

CROSS MATCHING

I = Incompatible
C = Compatible

To determine blood compatibility
for transfusion purposes,
recipient serum (plasma minus
fibrinogen) is mixed with the red
cells of various donors. If the
cells do not clump, a donor's
blood can be mixed with the
recipient's blood in a transfusion.

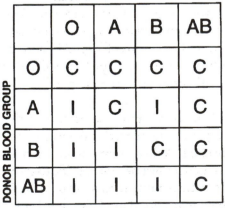

RECIPIENT BLOOD GROUP

		O	A	B	AB
	O	C	C	C	C
DONOR BLOOD GROUP	A	I	C	I	C
	B	I	I	C	C
	AB	I	I	I	C

In the early days of blood transfusion, Type O blood was considered the "universal donor," because there are no antigens on its red cell membrane. Type AB blood was considered the "universal recipient," because there are no antibodies (anti-A, anti-B) in its plasma. Today, the only time Type O is used is when a Type A or B or AB individual is in an emergency state and no other blood type is available.

universal donor

universal recipient

What happens when a Type A blood person receives Type B blood? He or she experiences what is known as a hemolytic transfusion reaction. This usually occurs when donor red cells and recipient plasma are incompatible. The more severe reactions in such a case may include shock, chills, fever, chest pain, dyspnea (shortness of breath), back pain, and/or abnormal bleeding. Death may also result. For an anesthetized patient, hypotension (low blood pressure) and evidence of disseminated intravascular coagulation (DIC) (See p. 78.) may be the first indications that the wrong blood type has been used. Administration of the wrong blood type is usually due to clerical error.

hemolytic transfusion reaction

DIC

The Rh Factor

The Rh factor of blood is another term associated with the ABO blood typing system. This factor is an antigen and was originally discovered in the Rhesus monkey, hence "Rh." The + or - sign used in conjunction with blood types A, B, AB, and O (e.g., A+, O-, AB+) indicates the presence or absence of the Rh factor on the red cell membrane. The positive sign indicates the presence and the minus sign the absence.

+ or -

The Rh factor, like the ABO blood, is type specific. A person must receive either Rh+ or Rh- blood, depending on his or her specific Rh factor. When an Rh- person receives Rh+ blood there may be few complications due to "incompatibility." However, a subsequent transfusion is potentially lethal because by then the

Figure 16 Rh NEGATIVE MOTHER WITH Rh POSITIVE FETUS

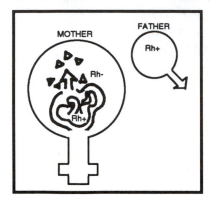

1. FIRST PREGNANCY

- NO HARM TO FETUS
- NO PROBLEMS FOR MOTHER

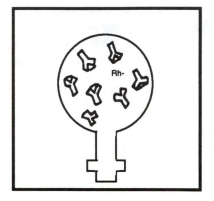

2. BEFORE AND AFTER DELIVERY OF
   FIRST CHILD

- MOTHER HAS DEVELOPED ANTIBODIES TO
  Rh+ FACTOR OF THE FETUS

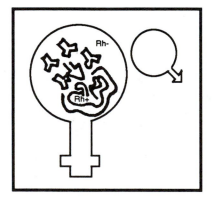

3. SECOND PREGNANCY

- MOTHER'S ANTIBODIES
  ATTACK FETAL BLOOD CELLS
- HDN OCCURS

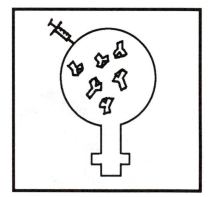

RhoGAM PREVENTS MOTHER'S
ANTIBODIES FROM FORMING

RhoGAM CAN BE ADMINISTERED:

- TO AN Rh- MOTHER WITH Rh+ HUSBAND
- ANY TIME THERE IS A MIX OF BLOOD
  BETWEEN MOTHER AND FETUS (e.g.,
  ECTOPIC PREGNANCY,
  MISCARRIAGE, AMNIOCENTESIS)
- TO A WOMAN OF CHILDBEARING AGE
- TO AN RH- WOMAN NEEDING Rh+ PLATELETS
- AFTER EACH Rh+ CHILD

recipient has developed antibodies for Rh+ blood from the previous transfusion. The result can be a severe immune reaction. For example, an A- patient may receive A+ blood with few complications, but another A+ transfusion is dangerous. That is because antibodies developed from the previous transfusion destroy the new blood that is being transfused.

A commonly used example to illustrate the significance of the Rh factor is an Rh- mother and an Rh+ father who have a baby that is Rh+. (See Figure 16.) In this case, any fetal blood that leaks across the placenta stimulates the mother's immune system to make antibodies against the Rh+ blood of the fetus. With the first child there is usually no problem, but in later pregnancies an Rh+ fetus is in jeopardy because the antibodies produced by the mother in the first pregnancy will attack the blood of the next fetus and may cause a condition known as hemolytic disease of the newborn (HDN). Fetal death may be prevented by an exchange transfusion. Doctors can now prevent this threat by giving the mother an injection called RhoGAM (Rh immune globulin). RhoGAM neutralizes antibodies produced against the Rh antigen.

RhoGAM

There is no problem when an Rh+ mother has an Rh- fetus. The mother has the antibodies in her plasma but the fetus's blood has no antigens (Rh factor) to stimulate the mother's immune system.

1. How are blood types identified?

2. Define antigen.

3. What is the blood type that corresponds to each of the following:
   1. neither antigen
   2. antigens A and B
   3. A antigen
   4. B antigen

4. Define antibody.

5. What two antibodies appear in blood and are used in blood typing? In what portion of the blood do they appear?

6. Neither antibody agglutinates Type O blood cells. Why?

7. What antibodies correspond to each of the following blood types?
   1. Type A blood
   2. Type B blood
   3. Type AB blood
   4. Type O blood

8. When is universal type O blood administered?

9. What is meant by hemolytic transfusion reaction?

10. True or false. HDN results in the first pregnancy of an Rh- mother with an Rh+ baby.

11. What is the name of the immune globulin given to an Rh- mother to neutralize antibodies produced against the Rh antigen of the fetus?

5   RED BLOOD CELLS (ERYTHROCYTES)

Red Blood Cell Formation

When red blood cells (RBCs) mature they receive a full complement of hemoglobin (Hgb) and also undergo condensation of the nucleus. (See Glossary.) As the red cells ready themselves for expulsion from the bone marrow into the circulation, the endothelial lining of the capillary in the bone marrow develops a pore or opening. The red cell squeezes through the pore, whereupon the nucleus is pinched off. The enucleated mature RBCs are released from the marrow into the circulation and have a life span of approximately 120 days.

Unlike most cells of the body, mature RBCs, once in the circulation, do not contain a nucleus. There are two reasons for this. 1)The main function of a red blood cell is the transport of oxygen and carbon dioxide, therefore, the presence of a nucleus would decrease the amount of space available to these gases. 2)The nucleus of a cell has a certain mass or weight, therefore, "nucleated" RBCs in the body would add significantly to the weight of the blood and increase the workload of the heart by about 20 percent. Such adaptations have contributed to the development of an efficient human body.

The Main Function of Red Cells

The primary function of red cells is the transport of oxygen and carbon dioxide. This process is made possible by a chemically complex protein molecule present in the red cell called hemoglobin, or Hgb. (See Figure 17, p. 34). During circulation through the lungs, Hgb becomes almost fully saturated with oxygen, making the blood bright red. As RBCs perfuse the capillary beds of tissues and organs, oxygen is released from hemoglobin to the tissues.

hemoglobin/ Hgb

33

Figure 17 STRUCTURE OF Hgb

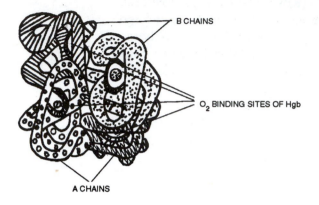

B CHAINS

O_2 BINDING SITES OF Hgb

A CHAINS

Figure 18 ALVEOLAR CAPILLARY NETWORK

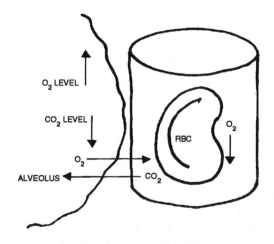

O_2 LEVEL

CO_2 LEVEL

O_2

RBC

O_2

O_2

ALVEOLUS

CO_2

The transfer of O_2 and CO_2 takes place at the alveolar capillary network of the lung.

In the red cells of normal adults, Hgb consists of two alpha (A) and two beta (B) chains, with a heme molecule attached to each chain. These chains consist of amino acids, which are the building blocks of proteins. The heme molecule attached to each chain is responsible for the red color of blood. Hgb biosynthesis (production) takes place in a cellular structure of the red blood cell known as the mitochondria. When the mature red cell enters the circulation from the bone marrow it loses the mitochondria as well as the nucleus.

heme molecule

The concentration of Hgb in a patient is a matter of concern, because Hgb's main function is the transport of oxygen from the lungs to the tissues and the transport of carbon dioxide in the reverse direction. Healthy patient physiology depends on the oxygen-transport capability of the blood. (See Figures 18 and 19.)

An accurate indication of the oxygen-carrying capacity of blood can be taken by measuring the concentration of Hgb. (See Appendix.) When Hgb concentration is low, tissues may not receive an adequate amount of oxygen, and over time this presents problems. Poor oxygen tissue perfusion results in poor healing of tissue and can also cause an increased workload on the heart, among other complications.

poor tissue perfusion

Figure 19 OXYGEN-CARBON DIOXIDE TRANSFER

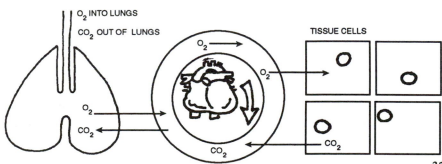

The oxygen that tissues receive depends on three factors: 1) the amount of blood flow to the tissues, 2) the level of Hgb concentration in the blood, and 3) the affinity of Hgb for oxygen. If any one of these is abnormal, the body automatically compensates by altering one or both of the others. For example, if the Hgb concentration is low, the body compensates by automatically increasing the heart rate, which in turn increases the amount of blood delivered to the tissues. Patients with an abnormality of one of the factors undergo an adjustment in one or both of the other two in order that optimal tissue perfusion (oxygenation) be maintained.

optimal tissue perfusion (oxygenation)

affinity of Hgb for oxygen

The affinity of Hgb for oxygen is regulated by three intracellular factors: 1) hydrogen ion concentration, or pH; 2) carbon dioxide; and 3) the chemical 2,3-diphosphoglycerate (2,3-DPG). If one of these three factors is not within its normal limits, Hgb will not release oxygen as readily to the tissues. (See Normal Values in Appendix.)

The Role of 2,3-Diphosphoglycerate (2,3-DPG)

Another important chemical found in red cells is 2,3-DPG. This molecule is present in the same concentration as Hgb in the blood and is bound to Hgb. The function of 2,3-DPG is to lower Hgb's affinity for oxygen so that Hgb releases oxygen to the tissues more easily. Without 2,3-DPG, Hgb would release little oxygen to the tissues.

stored blood and 2,3-DPG

The discovery of the role of 2,3-DPG in oxygen release to tissues has provided clinical medicine with new insights about stored blood. Stored blood has very low levels of 2,3-DPG. This is a serious situation for patients receiving large volumes of stored blood, because the amount of oxygen released to the tissues is then minimal. Transfused cells depleted of 2,3-DPG can regain only half their normal level back in a 24-

hour period, and this may not be rapid enough for a patient already compromised or severely ill. Adding 2,3-DPG to stored blood is of little value because the red cell membrane is impermeable (will not allow in) to this molecule. It has been shown that 2,3-DPG is an important regulator of Hgb function. The chemical 2,3-DPG allows Hgb to release oxygen to the tissues more easily.

The Shape of Red Cells

RBCs are flexible, biconcave discs with a diameter of 7 microns (μ) and a thickness of 2 microns. (See Appendix.) This shape allows the red cell to have a maximum surface area and thus facilitates the transfer of gases into and out of the cell. Its flexibility also enables a RBC easily to undergo the changes in shape necessary for travel through the capillaries of the body.

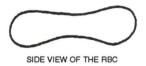

SIDE VIEW OF THE RBC

The Number of Red Cells

The number of red cells in the average adult is 4.5-5.5 x 10^6/mm^3. (The average number of blood cells is usually 5,000,000 per cubic millimeter of blood for males and 4,500,000 for females.) This number is standard, and any deviation from it suggests a problem. If there are too many RBCs in the circulation or a high RBC cell count exists, the condition is referred to as polycythemia. It is often seen in patients with cyanotic heart disease.

polycythemia

A high RBC number presents circulatory problems for the patient; the blood is so thick that it blocks the microvasculature of the lungs and kidneys. A low RBC count is termed anemia and is often seen in patients receiving chemotherapy or radiation therapy for bone

37

Figure 20 RBC PRODUCTION / ERYTHROPOIETIN PRODUCTION

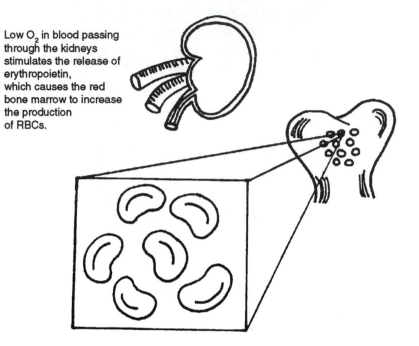

Low O$_2$ in blood passing
through the kidneys
stimulates the release of
erythropoietin,
which causes the red
bone marrow to increase
the production
of RBCs.

Figure 21 HEMATOCRITS

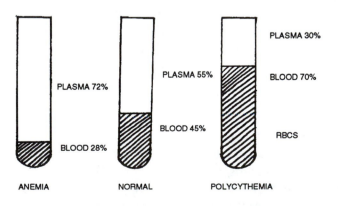

PLASMA 72%

BLOOD 28%

ANEMIA

PLASMA 55%

BLOOD 45%

NORMAL

PLASMA 30%

BLOOD 70%

RBCS

POLYCYTHEMIA

tumors. Anemia indicates there are not enough red cells in the circulation to transport sufficient amounts of oxygen to the tissues. With anemia other body systems have to compensate to deliver an adequate amount of oxygen to the tissues. For example, the heart beats faster and breathing becomes more rapid as the lungs take in air.

anemia

The Role of Erythropoietin

The production of RBCs is termed erythropoiesis. It is initiated by a hormone called erythropoietin, which is produced and released by the kidneys and circulated in the plasma. When a person's Hgb level is below normal, which can happen a number of ways, the tissues do not receive enough oxygen. This condition is called hypoxia. In hypoxia the kidneys are stimulated to increase the production of erythropoietin, which activates the stem cells in the marrow to produce more RBCs. (See Figure 20.)

erythropoiesis

hypoxia

The Hematocrit

An important factor in red cell physiology is the hematocrit (Hct), or percentage of whole blood occupied by the formed elements. The Hct is considered to be an index of the red cell concentration and thus an indirect measure of the oxygen-carrying capacity of the blood. In the normal adult, the Hct is between 38-45%. This indicates that 38-45% of the whole blood is made up of red cells. Remember, WBCs and platelets make up only 1% of the Hct.

Hct

The Hct and Hgb are related: the Hct is approximately three times the value of the Hgb. For example, if a patient's Hgb is 15 g/dl (grams per deciliter), then the Hct should be about 45%. When the formed elements make up 45% of the blood, then the other 55% consists of plasma. (See Figure 21.) A unit of stored homologous RBCs elevates the Hct by about 3-4%. For example, if the Hct is 35%, a unit of RBCs raises it to 38%.

39

Hemodilution

IVs or crystalloids

As the name suggests, hemodilution means "to dilute the blood." This usually occurs when intravenous solutions (IVs) or crystalloids are administered. These solutions are used to replace lost fluids or to keep veins open. Examples of IV solutions are Normal Saline, Dextrose, Lactated Ringers, etc.

normovolemic anemia

Hemodilution is accomplished before surgery if the medical team expects the patient to lose a lot of blood. Some of the patient's blood is removed and replaced with crystalloid. (See Figure 22.) This is called normovolemic anemia. The theory is that the patient loses less blood during surgery if there are fewer red cells in the circulation. After surgery the team reinfuses the blood that was removed prior to surgery in order to elevate the Hct of the patient.

Hemodilution is used in cardiac surgery. The heart-lung machine is a pump that must be primed (crystalloids added) with about 2200 ccs (cubic centimeters) of crystalloid solution. When the procedure utilizing

Figure 22 PATIENT UNDERGOING HEMODILUTION

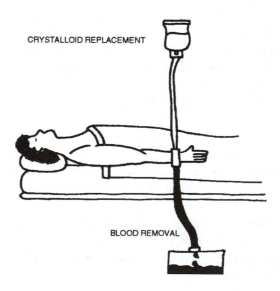

CRYSTALLOID REPLACEMENT

BLOOD REMOVAL

the pump begins, the 2200 ccs of fluid enters the patient's vascular space and reduces the Hct to about 20-25%.

During a bypass procedure, hemodilution has a number of advantages. 1) Hemodiluted blood is less viscous and flows more easily, resulting in better tissue perfusion. In bypass, patients are also cooled down to about 28°C, further easing hemodiluated blood flow. 2) Hemodilution increases capillary perfusion. 3) Because so much homologous blood is needed to prime the heart-lung machine during surgery, hemodilution prevents the patient from being exposed to unnecessary disease transmission through the use of homologous blood.

The absolute minimum that blood should be hemodiluted to is 15%. The amount of crystalloid fluid used during bypass is not really a concern because the patient is given drugs to help diurese (make urine) a major portion of this fluid.

Figure 23 RED BLOOD CELL HEMOLYSIS

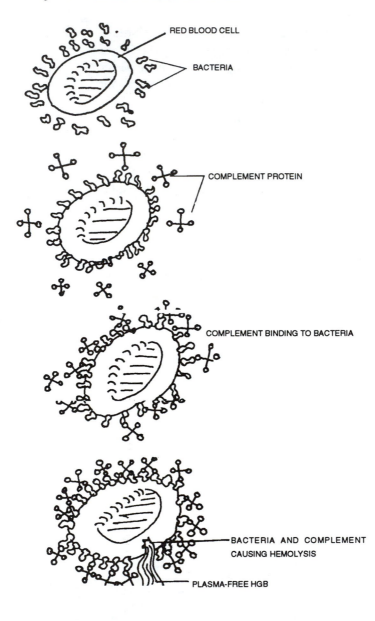

RED BLOOD CELL

BACTERIA

COMPLEMENT PROTEIN

COMPLEMENT BINDING TO BACTERIA

BACTERIA AND COMPLEMENT
CAUSING HEMOLYSIS

PLASMA-FREE HGB

Red Cell Hemolysis

Hemolysis refers to the destruction of the red cell membrane and is a serious problem. (See Figure 23.) It may be caused by a number of factors: 1) the immune response; for example, when a unit of the wrong type of blood is administered; 2) sepsis (bacterial or viral infection), which can cause the red cells to hemolyze; and 3) red cell membrane stress caused by high suction pressure during autologous blood recovery, with the use of a cardiac bypass pump, or by the hemodialysis machine, etc.

As red blood cells age their membranes become fragile and more easily hemolyzed. Older cells near the end of their life cycle are normally removed by the spleen, which is an organ located in the upper left-hand corner of the abdomen. Hemolyzed cells, from whatever cause, can present problems to patients. When the cell ruptures Hgb is released, a condition called plasma-free Hgb. In this case, Hgb can no longer transport oxygen, so the blood's ability to oxygenate tissue is decreased. The cell stroma (remnant of the ruptured cell) may block the microvasculature of the lung and kidneys causing these organs to fail.

plasma-free Hgb

RED BLOOD CELLS / QUESTIONS

1. What is the term used for red blood cells?

2. Where are red blood cells formed?

3. What is their approximate life span?

4. Describe the main function of RBCs.

5. What is the name of the complex protein molecule present in red blood cells? Its abbreviation?

6. Describe the role hemoglobin plays in getting oxygen to tissues.

7. Why is blood the color red?

8. Explain why normal patient physiology depends on Hgb.

9. What three factors contribute to optimal tissue perfusion (oxygenation) vital for patient health?

10. Under what circumstances and why does the physician order stored blood to return Hgb to a normal level?

11. How does stored blood elevate the Hgb?

12. What role does 2,3-DPG play in the release of oxygen to the tissues?

13. What problem may be posed to a seriously ill patient who receives a lot of stored blood?

14. The shape of a red blood cell is significant. Give one reason why.

15. Polycythemia and anemia are terms associated with the number of red blood cells in the circulation. Describe the implications of each to the patient.

16. What is the condition called when too little oxygen is in the tissues?

17. What physiological event is stimulated by hypoxia?

18. Give a definition of the hematocrit.

19. What are formed elements?

20. How is the Hct used?

21. What does it mean for average adults if the Hct is between 38-45%?

22. True or False. The Hct is approximately ten times the value of the Hgb.

23. What does the term hemodilution mean?

24. Describe two circumstances in which a patient may undergo hemodilution.

25. There are several advantages to hemodilution during cardiac surgery. Describe two.

26. What does the term hemolysis mean?

27. Describe two causes of hemolysis.

28. When the cell ruptures Hgb is released. What problems occur?

6 WHITE BLOOD CELLS (LEUKOCYTES)

White blood cells (WBCs), or leukocytes, are blood cells that circulate throughout the body and tissues providing protection against foreign organisms and matter.

To carry out their intended function, WBCs must be highly mobile. They must be able to squeeze through pores in the capillaries and move into the tissues, a property known as diapedesis. When a foreign organism enters the body it releases a chemical substance that stimulates the WBCs and causes them to be attracted to the area of invasion. This process is known as chemotaxis. It plays an important role in WBCs function in the immune system. (See Figure 24.)

WBCs are divided into three groups: the granulocytes, monocytes, and lymphocytes. Granulocytes are named for the granules that are present in their cytoplasm (the jelly-like substance found within the cell). They are divided further into neutrophils, eosinophils, and basophils. After they leave the circulatory system and enter the tissues, monocytes become macrophages. The lymphocytes are divided into T cells and B cells. Each WBC has a specific function in the immune response.

diapedesis

chemotaxis

WBCs
1.   2.
Granulocytes   Monocytes
neutrophils   ▼
eosinophils   macrophages
basophils

3.
Lymphocytes
T cells
B cells

Figure 24 CHEMOTAXIS AND DIAPEDESIS

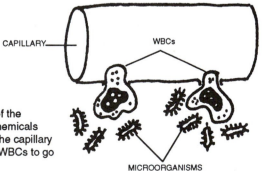

CAPILLARY

WBCs

Antigens on the surface of the microorganism release chemicals (chemotaxis) that cause the capillary pores to dilate and allow WBCs to go through (diapedesis).

MICROORGANISMS

The Number of White Blood Cells

The average adult male has 75 trillion white blood cells (7,000 per cubic millimeter). The normal WBC count in a sample of blood from an adult is 5,000-10,000/mm³. When an infection occurs in the body the WBC level of the blood increases, for example to 16,000/mm³ or higher, depending on the length of time the infection has been present. An increased WBC count is a classic sign of infection somewhere in the body.

Granulocytes: Neutrophils, Eosinophils, Basophils

Neutrophils

Like other blood cells, neutrophils develop in the bone marrow. Their life cycle, which takes place in the marrow, blood, and tissues, is short, and in some instances lasts only a few hours. When neutrophils mature and enter the circulation 50% of them circulate in the blood and 50% adhere to the blood vessel walls. Neutrophils move freely between the blood and the tissues of the body where they carry out their primary function; namely, to engulf foreign organisms

Figure 25 PHAGOCYTOSIS

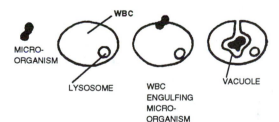

MICRO-
ORGANISM

WBC

LYSOSOME

WBC
ENGULFING
MICRO-
ORGANISM

VACUOLE

LYSOME READY
TO RELEASE
HYDROLYTIC
ENZYMES INTO
VACUOLE
CONTAINING
MICRO-
ORGANISM

DIGESTED
MICRO-
ORGANISM
IN VACUOLE

DIGESTED
MICRO-
ORGANISM

that they encounter. This process is called phagocytosis. (See Figure 25.)

In the presence of inflammation, neutrophils, attracted by chemicals, continually move into an infected area, phagocytize, die, and are themselves phagocytized by macrophages. Neutrophils are generally the first cells to enter an infected area, followed by monocytes. Neutrophils continue their attack until all foreign material has been engulfed.

Eosinophils

Eosinophils are produced and mature in bone marrow. They appear at sites where foreign protein and parasites are found and in association with allergic reactions. The number of eosinophils increases in these situations, but only in small numbers, making them difficult to study. They are armed with binding sites for IgE and IgG immunoglobulins as well as complement proteins. They are specifically designed to phagocytize cells coated with IgG, IgE, and complement. Eosinophils prefer tissue residence rather than living in the circulation. They live in the skin, lungs, and airways (bronchi and bronchioles) of the lungs.

Basophils

Basophils, produced in the marrow, are the least common of all granulocytes. They exhibit chemotaxis and some phagocytic activity. Their main function, it is believed, is to release heparin (an anticoagulant) in areas of foreign matter invasion to prevent blood from clotting. If blood clots in the area of invasion, WBCs cannot reach the organisms to destroy them and the tissue necroses (dies). Basophils also release histamine in the area of invasion. Histamine causes the blood vessels to dilate their pores. Other granulocytes can then leave the circulation more easily and enter the tissues.

Monocytes/Macrophages

Monocytes are produced in bone marrow, but unlike other cells in the circulation are considered to be immature. When a monocyte leaves the blood it travels to the tissue. Once in the tissue it spends most of its time maturing into a macrophage, while at the same time being actively phagocytic.

As the monocyte develops into a macrophage there is an increase in the number of intracellular (within the cell) lysosomes. Lysosomes are membrane-bound vacuoles (little sacs found in the cytoplasm of cells) containing enzymes. These enzymes allow the macrophage to "digest" the foreign matter that it engulfs. Macrophages are scattered throughout the body, most commonly lining the sinusoids (spaces) in the liver, spleen, and lungs.

lysosomes

Lymphocytes

Lymphocytes are most easily understood in conjunction with the immune response. They are also the most complex of the WBCs. When stimulated by antigens, lymphocytes produce a number of different cell types. Lymphocytes known as T and B cells initiate responses of the immune system. They are designed to neutralize or destroy foreign material. (See Figure 26.)

When a virus or bacteria invades the body the immune response is stimulated. The body recognizes foreign matter as not "self" and sends neutrophils and macrophages to engulf it. As the macrophage attacks a foreign invader it displays specific markers on its surface. These markers are antigens that signal T cells to go into action. When T cells become stimulated they release a chemical that activates the B cells. The B cells in turn divide and mature into plasma cells that produce antibodies. Antibodies either stop the invader or make the invader more vulnerable to neutrophils.

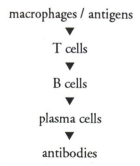

macrophages / antigens
▼
T cells
▼
B cells
▼
plasma cells
▼
antibodies

Lymphocytes also play a role when the body rejects a transplanted organ. Antigens on the donor organ are recognized by the host lymphocytes as foreign. The host B cells produce antibodies in response to the foreign tissue and destroy it. Conversely, a transplanted organ can be the culprit; its lymphocytes may recognize the host as foreign and mount an attack against it. In both cases, similar processes are involved and the result is organ rejection. This is why patients who have had organ transplants must have their immune system suppressed with drugs.

Figure 26 LYMPHOCYTE DIFFERENTIATION

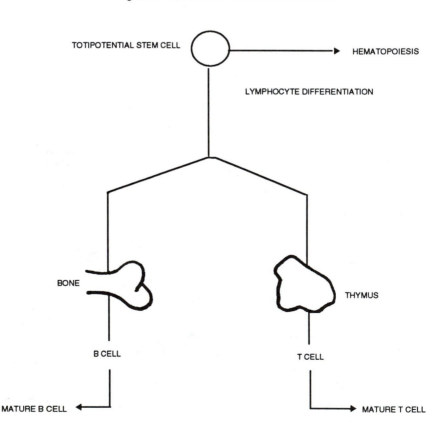

T Cells and B Cells

There are two functional classes of lymphocytes: the T cells and B cells. Both are produced in the bone marrow. T cells complete maturation in the thymus, a gland that lies on the heart and atrophies with age. The thymus confers on the T cells the ability to recognize antigens and control antibody production. T cells are directly involved with cellular immunity. Receptors on their surface enable them to recognize specific antigens. On recognizing an antigen, T cells stimulate B cells to produce an antibody specifically for that antigen.

B cells are released from bone marrow and reside in the lymph nodes, which are conglomerations of lymphatic tissue found throughout the body, most noticeably in the armpits and groin. B cells, when stimulated or activated by T cells, mature into plasma cells, the cells directly responsible for antibody production. B cells/ plasma cells are involved only in antibody production.

thymus

lymph nodes

WHITE BLOOD CELLS / QUESTIONS

1. What is the term used for white blood cells?

2. What is the name of the chemical process that stimulates WBCs to the area of foreign invasion? a. Diapedesis b. Chemotaxis c. Hemolysis

3. Name the two kinds of lymphocytes.

4. What does an increased level of WBCs indicate?

5. What is the primary function of neutrophils?

6. What two chemicals are released by basophils?

7. Where are eosinophils found?

8. What WBC is believed to release the anticoagulant heparin?

9. Why is it essential that clotting not take place in an infected area?

10. What WBC develops into a macrophage?

11. Macrophages contain membrane-bound vacuoles of enzymes called lysosomes. What is the function of lysosomes?

12. Lymphocytes are a complex WBC. Stimulated by antigens, they produce different types of cells and initiate immune responses carried out by T and B cells. What role do they play in organ transplant rejection?

13. The lymphatic system works in conjunction with the blood-vascular system. How do B cells demonstrate this?

7 PLATELETS

Platelets, or thrombocytes, are small, colorless, enucleated bodies. They are produced in the bone marrow by fragmentation of megakaryocytes. Megakaryocytes are large cells found in bone marrow that produce platelets by fragmenting their cytoplasm. Platelets play a vital role in the hemostatic process, which prevents blood loss. (See below.) When the endothelial lining of a blood vessel is traumatized, platelets are stimulated to go to the site of injury, where they form a plug that helps reduce blood loss.

The normal platelet count in an adult is 150,000 - 400,000/mm^3 (250,000 per cubic millimeter). When the platelet count increases the condition is known as thrombocytosis. This may occur in certain disease states such as cancer, chronic infections, and certain blood diseases. It may cause increased blood clot formation. When the platelet count decreases a condition called thrombocytopenia occurs. This may happen either as a result of decreased platelet production (e.g., bone tumor, chemotherapy) or excessive platelet destruction (e.g., transfusion reaction, immune response). Platelets range in size from 2-4 microns (μ), but in certain situations can be as large as 25-40 microns. Once platelets are released into the circulatory system they have a life span of 9-12 days. Young platelets are more effective in achieving and maintaining hemostasis. Old, damaged, and nonfunctional platelets are removed by the spleen.

The Role of Platelets in Hemostasis

Hemostasis is the process carried out by the body to maintain blood in the vascular system. When blood is lost the body provides platelets and a network of chemicals that function to prevent blood loss by forming a fibrin clot at the site of the damage. Coagulation, or blood clotting, refers to the process in which platelets interact with coagulation proteins.

PLATELETS / QUESTIONS

1.   What is another name for platelets?

2.   True or False. Platelets are formed elements.

3.   Describe the chief function of platelets.

4.   What do platelets do when the endothelial lining of a blood vessel is damaged?

5.   What happens to nonfunctional platelets?

6.   Define hemostasis and the role of platelets in it.

8   PLASMA

Plasma is the liquid portion of blood in which the formed elements are suspended. It is a straw-colored, viscous solution comprised of solids (proteins, electrolytes, hormones, and vitamins) and water. The solids are dissolved in the plasma. They are in continuous communication with the interstitial fluid (fluid that bathes the cells outside the vascular system) via the capillary pores (spaces in the capillary wall that allow substances to pass through).

interstitial fluid

capillary pores

Plasma contains many substances (e.g., proteins, electrolytes, and hormones) that are in continuous communication with the tissues of the body. However, some of plasma's substances, such as proteins, cannot pass easily through the capillary pores due to their large size. The great majority of them stay in the vascular space where they exert colloid osmotic pressure, or oncotic pressure. It is this pressure that maintains fluid in the vascular space. Osmotic pressure pulls water from the interstitial space into the capillary so that equilibrium can be maintained on either side of the capillary wall. (See Figure 27.)

colloid osmotic pressure, or oncotic pressure

Proteins in plasma may also be used by the body tissues when proteins obtained from food do not provide for normal body needs. Plasma proteins, along with certain electrolytes, also contribute to the buffering capacity of the blood. Buffering is a term used to describe the body's ability to regulate the pH of blood. (The pH describes the acidity or alkalinity of a solution. If acidic, pH is low, between 1-7; if basic, pH is high, between 7-14. Numbers 1-7 and 7-14 are logarithmic measurements.) The normal range of blood pH is 7.35-7.45, slightly basic.

buffering
pH

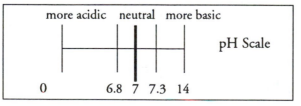

pH Scale

more acidic   neutral   more basic

0   6.8 7 7.3   14

Figure 27   FUNCTIONS OF PLASMA

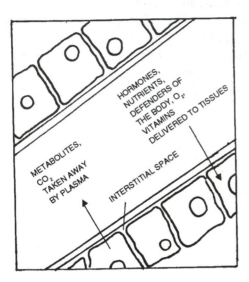

Transport of substances to and from tissues

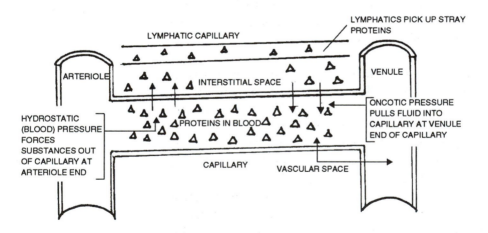

Plasma components as they diffuse through a capillary

If the pH of blood changes, either becoming more acidic or basic, there can be serious complications for the patient. For example, in acidosis, carbon dioxide (CO_2) or organic acids build up in the blood causing it to become acidic. The lungs and the kidneys control the level of acidosis. If acidosis is not controlled, the recovery or health of the patient can be compromised because blood and tissue physiology are no longer normal.

acidosis

The Electrolytes and Glucose in Plasma

The electrolytes in plasma function in a number of ways. An electrolyte is a chemical molecule that produces ions (See Glossary.) when placed in a solution such as water or plasma (which is basically water). Normal concentrations of electrolytes are essential for physiologic processes, e.g., nerve conduction and muscle contraction.

The main electrolytes in plasma are:

electrolytes

Sodium (Na^+), with a normal concentration of 138 - 148 mM/L

(mM/L means millimoles per liter of solution. The term *mole* is a measure of the gram molecular weight of a substance.)

Potassium (K^+) 3.5 - 5.2 mM/L

Calcium (Ca^{++}) 8.5 - 10.5 mM/L

Chlorine (Cl^-) 98 - 111 mM/L

Calcium, sodium, and potassium are necessary for normal impulse conduction in nerve and muscle fibers. Sodium plays an essential role in maintaining normal fluid balance within the cells of the body. If the sodium concentration is too high or too low, then the fluid balance shifts, with the cells either retaining or losing too much fluid.

57

glucose

insulin

Plasma also contains glucose (sugar), an essential source of energy for all tissues of the body. The normal concentration of glucose is 72 - 137 mg/dl (milligrams per deciliter). Sugar is dissolved in plasma and must get into the cell in order to supply energy to the cell. Sugar enters the red blood cell by the simple process of diffusion. Insulin, a hormone produced in the pancreas, allows sugar to penetrate other cells' membranes. Diabetics, people who lack the ability to produce insulin, must take insulin from other sources, such as insulin injection.

PLASMA / QUESTIONS

1. Give a one-sentence definition of plasma.

2. Describe one characteristic of plasma.

3. What is the fluid that bathes cells outside the vascular system?
    a. plasma   b. electrolytes
    c. interstitial fluid

4. True or False. Another term for the circulatory system is the vascular space.

5. The pH of blood is slightly basic. In acidosis does carbon dioxide or organic acids cause the blood to become more basic or more acidic?

6. What happens if blood pH becomes either more acidic or more basic?

7. What electrolyte in plasma is essential to maintain normal fluid balance in cells?
    a. potassium b. calcium c. sodium

8. What is the role of glucose in plasma?

9. What is the function of insulin?

9 HEMOSTASIS

The term hemostasis refers to the prevention of blood loss through processes that inhibit blood flow from a ruptured vessel. The hemostatic processes include: 1) vascular spasm, 2) platelet function, and 3) blood coagulation, or clotting. When a blood vessel is injured or damaged the hemostatic processes repair the break and stop the bleeding. (See Figure 28.)

vascular spasm
▼
platelet plug
▼
coagulation cascade
▼
fibrin clot

The first and most immediate hemostatic response to blood vessel injury is vascular spasm, a rapid constriction of the vessel. The second response is the formation of a platelet plug. The final response is the initiation of the coagulation cascade. (See p.66.) Together, all the responses help prevent blood loss by forming fibrin, the end step in the clotting process that holds the clot together.

clot lysis

Once a clot has formed and the vessel has repaired itself, a process known as clot lysis (lysis: to break) must occur so that normal blood flow through the vessel can resume. Coagulation and lysis work in conjunction with each other, but must be considered separately.

Figure 28 MECHANISMS OF COAGULATION

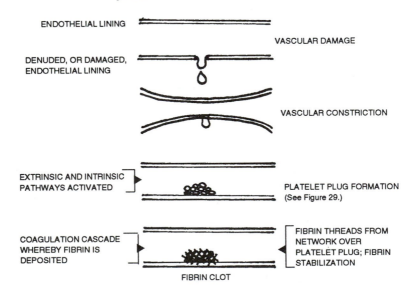

ENDOTHELIAL LINING

VASCULAR DAMAGE

DENUDED, OR DAMAGED, ENDOTHELIAL LINING

VASCULAR CONSTRICTION

EXTRINSIC AND INTRINSIC PATHWAYS ACTIVATED

PLATELET PLUG FORMATION
(See Figure 29.)

COAGULATION CASCADE WHEREBY FIBRIN IS DEPOSITED

FIBRIN THREADS FROM NETWORK OVER PLATELET PLUG; FIBRIN STABILIZATION

FIBRIN CLOT

Figure 29 MECHANISMS OF PLATELET ACTION

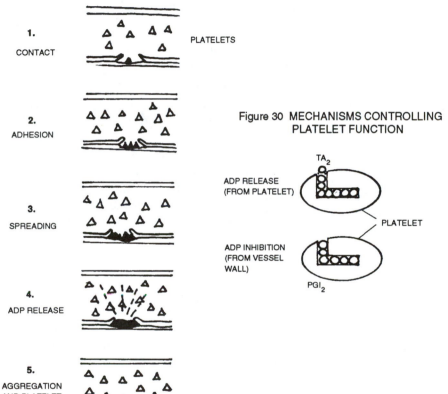

1.

CONTACT

PLATELETS

2.

ADHESION

Figure 30 MECHANISMS CONTROLLING
PLATELET FUNCTION

TA_2

ADP RELEASE
(FROM PLATELET)

PLATELET

3.

SPREADING

ADP INHIBITION
(FROM VESSEL
WALL)

PGI_2

4.

ADP RELEASE

5.

AGGREGATION
AND PLATELET
PLUG FORMATION

Vascular Spasm

The first response to vessel injury is vascular spasm. Vessel walls have smooth muscle fibers located within their structure that constrict to reduce the loss of blood. Other events occur in vascular spasm, such as edema (tissue swelling), chemical release, and shunting (the redirection of blood flow to nearby vessels).

edema
shunting

Arteries have thick walls and cannot control their bleeding by vascular spasm, platelet plug formation, or by coagulation proteins forming a clot. They must be repaired surgically in order to control bleeding.

Platelet Function in Coagulation

Platelets perform two functions in the hemostatic process. First, they form a plug that covers the break in the endothelial lining. Second, once the plug is formed, the platelet membrane provides the surface on which the activated coagulation proteins (clotting factors) bind. The active surface of the platelet is made possible by the presence of a phospholipid (chemically complex fat molecule). This phospholipid is called platelet factor 3, or PF-3.

PF-3

There are five steps involved in platelet interaction, or platelet plug formation, with a damaged vessel. (See Figure 29.) 1)The first step involves contact between the platelet and the damaged endothelial lining of the blood vessel. 2) In the second step, after contact has been made, the platelet adheres to the damaged surface. This is called adhesion. 3) Thereafter, the platelets spread out along the damaged surface changing shape (becoming flat) as they do. 4) The fourth step is release, in which platelets release a chemical called ADP (adenosine diphosphate). The release of ADP stimulates other platelets to aggregate to the area of damage. 5) The fifth and final step is called aggregation. Platelet plug

platelet plug formation
▼
contact
▼
adhesion
▼
spreading
▼
ADP release
▼
aggregation

formation provides an effective barrier to further blood loss. The platelet plug is formed by the interaction of the above steps, but the plug is only temporary. Coagulation proteins then take up their role to ensure hemostasis. (See p. 66.)

Prostaglandins Regulating ADP Release

ADP release is regulated by chemicals called prostaglandins. The most important ones are Thromboxane A_2 (TA_2) and Prostacyclin (PGI_2). They induce opposite effects. (See Figure 30.)

Thromboxane is synthesized (produced) in the platelet membrane and *increases* the amount of ADP released during platelet plug formation. PGI_2 is synthesized by the endothelial cells of the vessel wall and *decreases* ADP release. Thromboxane is released by the platelet membrane and results in the release of ADP, which causes platelets to aggregate to the area of injury. PGI_2 is released by the endothelial cells of the vessel so that ADP release is inhibited and platelets do not aggregate past the area of injury. Thromboxane and PGI_2 provide checks and balances in platelet aggregation. If there are not enough platelets at the site of injury, no plug forms. On the other hand, if too many platelets are present, blood flow through the vessel may be inhibited.

Because aspirin interferes with Thromboxane release it also blocks ADP release. Doctors often prescribe aspirin for older patients, as they say, "to help thin the blood." Aspirin does not thin the blood but does block Thromboxane, which prevents ADP release, which in turn prevents platelets from aggregating. Platelets that cannot aggregate cannot form a plug. The theory behind aspirin therapy is to prevent patients from forming clots to reduce their chances of having a stroke or TIA (transient ischemic attack), which is a "mini" stroke.

Thromboxane
Prostacyclin

PGI_2

63

Platelets and Foreign Surfaces

Foreign surfaces, such as vascular grafts, can interfere with hemostasis. A graft (synthetic material) does not synthesize Prostacyclin (PGI_2). However, graft insertion does stimulate platelet aggregation and platelets may aggregate beyond the endothelial wall damage and into the graft. This situation has the potential for causing graft thrombosis (obstruction of blood flow due to clot).

graft thrombosis

Platelets and Phospholipids

Once the platelet plug has formed over the area of injury the coagulation proteins, or clotting factors, are stimulated to react with a phospholipid (chemical). There are two types of phospholipids: 1) PF-3, a platelet membrane phospholipid, and 2) a tissue membrane phospholipid called tissue thromboplastin. (See Figure 31.) Each phospholipid is essential in the coagulation cascade, but occurs in different pathways, or series of events. Nature has provided two pathways (extrinsic and intrinsic) to prevent bleeding through clot formation. Both fully protect the patient from bleeding due either to vessel damage or to blood coming into contact with a foreign surface. (See p. 68.)

phospholipids:
1) PF-3, or platelet membrane
2) tissue membrane, or tissue thromboplastin

Figure 31 SOURCES OF PHOSPHOLIPIDS

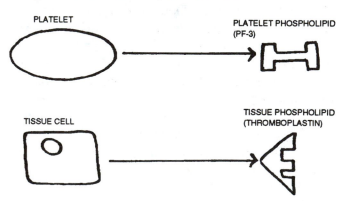

PLATELET

PLATELET PHOSPHOLIPID (PF-3)

TISSUE CELL

TISSUE PHOSPHOLIPID (THROMBOPLASTIN)

HEMOSTATIS / QUESTIONS

1. Explain what vascular spasm, platelet function, and blood coagulation have in common.

2. Which process occurs first in hemostasis? Describe what happens.

3. What is the end step in the hemostatic process?

4. For normal blood flow to occur after a clot has formed, what process must take place?

5. Write the correct version of this statement. Due to their thin walls arteries can control their bleeding by hemostasis and do not need to be repaired surgically.

6. Name the five steps in platelet plug formation.

7. Describe the role of ADP in platelet plug formation.

8. What are the chemicals that regulate ADP release called?

9. Match the correct word — plasma, Thromboxane, or PGI_2 — with the following:
    a. Causes platelets to aggregate to injury site
    b. Inhibits ADP release so platelets do not aggregate past the area of injury

10. What effect does aspirin have on platelet formation?

11. What are the two phospholipids involved in clotting and when are they activated?

10 THE COAGULATION CASCADE

The coagulation cascade is a complex system of actions and reactions among blood clotting factors. The coagulation cascade is also referred to as the enzyme cascade or protein cascade. The clotting factors are also referred to as coagulation factors, clotting proteins, coagulation proteins, or clotting enzymes, which are chemically designated as serine proteases.* Fibrin stabilization of the platelet plug, or formation of a fibrin clot, is the end product of the coagulation cascade. Coagulation factors circulate continuously in the blood and react when stimulated by a phospholipid. The coagulation cascade is initiated when phospholipids are released by activated platelets or injured tissue.

enzyme/protein/
coagulation cascade

coagulation cascade
▼
fibrin formation/
fibrin stabilization
of the platelet plug/
fibrin clot

phospholipids

The coagulation factors are listed below. They are referred to by Roman numerals, e.g., factor VI.

clotting factors are:
coagulation proteins/
cleavage enzymes/
serine proteases

I	Fibrinogen
II	Prothrombin
III	Platelet Factor-3 (Thromboplastin)
IV	Calcium
V	Labile Factor (Proaccelerin)
VI	Not Assigned
VII	Stable Factor (Proconvertin)
VIII	Antihemophiliac Factor A (AHF)
IX	Antihemophiliac Factor B (Christmas Factor)
X	Stuart-Prower Factor
XI	Antihemophiliac Factor C (PTA)
XII	Hageman Factor
XIII	Fibrin Stabilizing Factor (FSF)

The coagulation proteins form a cascade similar to a chain reaction. The reaction, however, does not occur in the sequential order suggested above. The numbers refer to the order in which the factors were discovered, not to the order in which they react to form a fibrin clot.

* Factors V and VIII are not serine proteases, but are commonly referred to as such.

In the coagulation cascade, molecules of activated clotting factors activate the next set of clotting factors in the chain reaction. Activation is achieved when factor, cleavage (splitting) enzymes, activate the next factors in the reaction by splitting off a piece of it. Whenever a piece of a factor is split off the factor is activated and then activates the next factor. All factors in the cascade are activated until fibrin is formed.

Cleavage enzymes are produced in the liver and circulate in the blood in high concentrations in the inactive form. If the enzymes were to circulate in the active form, fibrin would form everywhere and the coagulation factors would be very quickly consumed by the body. There would not be enough coagulation factors available for an event requiring coagulation. By circulating in the inactive form, cleavage enzymes prevent clot formation.

For clots to form, coagulation protein binding to phospholipids must occur. This binding is made possible by the availability of certain tissue or by platelet phospholipids and calcium. The presence of phospholipids is essential for clot formation. Coagulation factors circulating in the blood become activated only when exposed to tissue or platelet phospholipids. If phospholipids are not available, coagulation proteins cannot bind and no clot formation occurs. Platelet phospholipid is exposed (available) only from activated platelets. Tissue phospholipid is exposed only from damaged tissue.

coagulation proteins
bind to tissue or platelet
phospholipids
via a calcium bridge

▼

clot formation

Phospholipids bind coagulation proteins via a calcium bridge. Calcium is present in the plasma and is essential for normal coagulation. Tissue phospholipid binds only two chemicals, factor VII and calcium. Platelet phospholipid binds three, calcium and two factors. Phospholipids used in coagulation always bind calcium.

calcium bridge

In bank or autologous blood, chelating (binding) agents such as CPD and CPDA-1 are added to bind calcium and prevent clot formation. Chelating agents usually are

67

used as anticoagulants any time blood is collected for transfusions. Blood that clots is of no value to the patient.

rate limiting step

The rate limiting step (clot formation control) refers to the number and availability of clotting factors ready to bind with calcium and phospholipid. The ability of the body to form clots depends on the availability of clotting factors. If any clotting factor in the cascade is not available, a clot will not form, even if the cascade is initiated. Clotting factor deficiencies occur in diseases in which clotting factors are absent or not replenished, such as hemophilia or liver disease.

The Pathways of Coagulation

There are two pathways in the coagulation cascade that lead to fibrin formation and protect a person from bleeding. They are the intrinsic and extrinsic pathways. Each is activated by a different chemical, either platelet factor III or tissue thromboplastin. The pathways may be activated at the same time (as in surgery) or individually. Both pathways have in common a final pathway in which actions and reactions are identical. (See Figure 32.)

intrinsic and
extrinsic pathways

The intrinsic pathway is activated when blood is removed from the body or comes into contact with a foreign substance or surface, i.e., any nonendothelial surface. Examples of a nonendothelial surface include vascular graphs, surgical implants, and damaged endothelium. In the intrinsic pathway all factors necessary for clotting are available in the blood and clotting takes several minutes to occur.

The extrinsic pathway is activated when tissue is damaged and exposes tissue phospholipid. It is initiated by tissue injury, as in a cut, and by tissue thromboplastin, a substance that is extraneous to the blood. Clotting occurs within seconds and does not involve early coagulation reactions. During surgical procedures both the intrinsic and extrinsic pathways are stimulated because blood comes in contact with a foreign surface and tissue is cut.

Figure 32 COAGULATION CASCADE

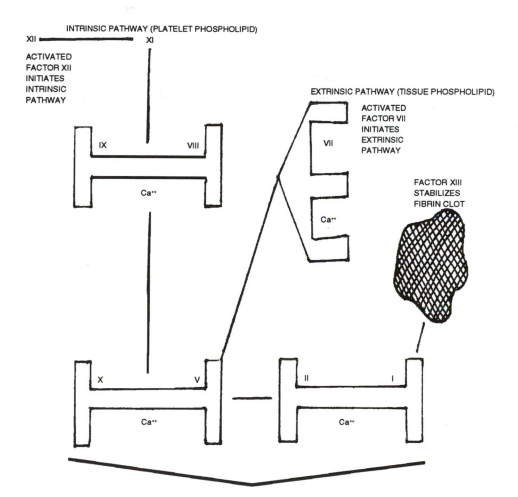

INTRINSIC PATHWAY (PLATELET PHOSPHOLIPID)

XII ━━━━━━━━━ XI

ACTIVATED
FACTOR XII
INITIATES
INTRINSIC
PATHWAY

EXTRINSIC PATHWAY (TISSUE PHOSPHOLIPID)

ACTIVATED
FACTOR VII
INITIATES
EXTRINSIC
PATHWAY

IX   VIII   VII

Ca⁺⁺   Ca⁺⁺

FACTOR XIII
STABILIZES
FIBRIN CLOT

X   V   II   I

Ca⁺⁺   Ca⁺⁺

FINAL COMMON PATHWAY

The Intrinsic Pathway

When an injured vessel exposes a surface denuded of its endothelial lining, a series of events is set in motion that leads to the formation of a fibrin clot. This series of events, referred to as the intrinsic pathway, begins intravascularly when the denuded endothelium activates factor XII. (See Figure 33.) Activated factor XIIa ("a" means activated) activates factor XI. Factor XIa activates factors IX and VIII, the first set of factors to bind to the platelet surface phospholipid (PF-3) via the calcium bridge. Factor IXa activates factors X and V, the second set of factors to bind to the platelet phospholipid.

PF-3

Factors V and VIII are not serine proteases like the other factors. They are known as "helper" factors, or co-enzymes. Unlike the serine proteases they circulate in the blood in the active form, are used once in coagulation, and are easily destroyed by the body. They are deficient in stored blood. Factors V and VIII are preserved, however, in fresh frozen plasma (FFP), which is obtained by removing the plasma from a unit of whole blood and then freezing it. Factor VIII in FFP may be used in the treatment of a certain type of hemophilia.

"helper" factors

The third set of factors to bind to the platelet phospholipid are factors II and I. They conclude the intrinsic pathway. Factor II (prothrombin) cleaves factor I, fibrinogen, into monomers (smaller units of fibrin). Activated by factor XIII, the monomers polymerize (form chains) to form a fibrin clot.

The Extrinsic Pathway

The extrinsic pathway involves tissue phospholipid (tissue thromboplastin) activation as the result of injury and leads to the formation of a fibrin clot. Just as a platelet provides a phospholipid for the intrinsic pathway, tissue provides the phospholipid for the ex-

Figure 33 INTRINSIC PATHWAY

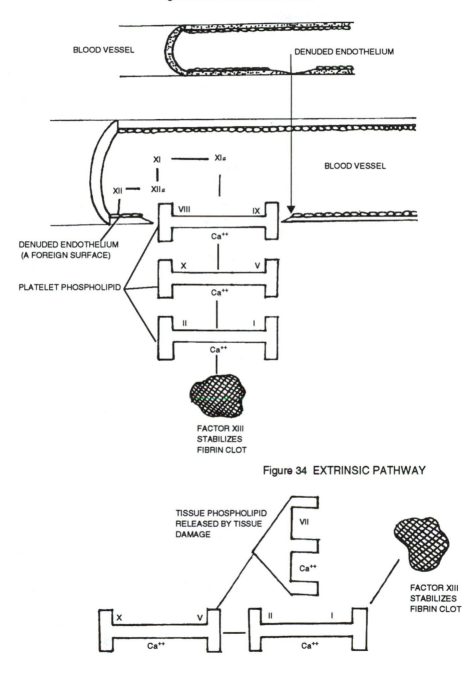

BLOOD VESSEL

DENUDED ENDOTHELIUM

BLOOD VESSEL

XI — XIa

XII — XIIa

VIII   IX

Ca^{++}

DENUDED ENDOTHELIUM
(A FOREIGN SURFACE)

PLATELET PHOSPHOLIPID

X   V

Ca^{++}

II   I

Ca^{++}

FACTOR XIII
STABILIZES
FIBRIN CLOT

Figure 34 EXTRINSIC PATHWAY

TISSUE PHOSPHOLIPID
RELEASED BY TISSUE
DAMAGE

VII

Ca^{++}

FACTOR XIII
STABILIZES
FIBRIN CLOT

X   V

Ca^{++}

II   I

Ca^{++}

trinsic pathway. Normally, tissue phospholipid is not present in blood, but is released at the time of tissue damage.

The extrinsic pathway binds factor VII and calcium. Activated factor VIIa activates factors X and V. (See Figure 34.) This point in the pathway is known as the "common pathway," because the intrinsic and extrinsic pathways share it. The production of fibrin is the result of either pathway.

Vitamin K and Coumadin

Vitamin K is a fat soluble vitamin essential for normal blood coagulation. Vitamin K allows the coagulation factors to bind to calcium. The coagulation factors that require Vitamin K are factors II, VII, IX, and X. These factors are often referred to as "Vitamin K-dependent factors." If the body is low or deficient in Vitamin K, normal coagulation cannot occur.

The drug Coumadin (chemical name: Warfarin) functions as an anticoagulant. It blocks the action of Vitamin K to prevent the coagulation factors from binding to calcium. Coumadin is used in the treatment of preventing blood clots, for people who have artificial heart valves, and for people susceptible to strokes.

Clot Lysis

Clot lysis (lysis: to break) is the dissolution of the blood clot in a vessel that has been injured and is healed. (See Figure 35.) It is nature's way of restoring normal blood flow to a vessel after injury. A damaged vessel forms a clot to prevent the loss of blood. After the vessel has healed the clot must be dissolved so that normal blood flow can return to the vessel. Clot lysis must occur slowly, for if the clot is dissolved too quickly, before adequate healing takes place, bleeding will resume.

Just as coagulation proceeds via either of two pathways, so clot lysis proceeds via either of two pathways. In the intrinsic pathway, plasminogen, a naturally occurring chemical found in the blood, is cleaved (split) to its active form, called plasmin, by the action of factor XIIa. In the extrinsic pathway, plasminogen is activated to plasmin by tissue plasminogen activators (TPA), which are normal substances produced by the tissues.

intrinsic and extrinsic pathways

plasminogen

plasmin

TPA

When shed blood is collected postoperatively by wound drainage from a patient who is bleeding rapidly, clots appear in the collection reservoir. The blood that is being shed does not have time to react with tissue plasminogen activators (TPA), which is why the clots appear in the collection system. On the other hand, if blood loss occurs slowly, clots are not found in the reservoir because the blood has had time to react with tissue plasminogen activators (TPA).

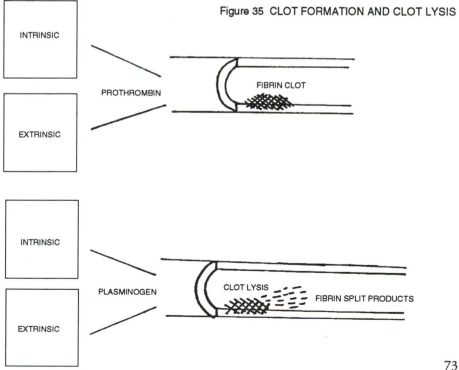

Figure 35 CLOT FORMATION AND CLOT LYSIS

Fibrin Split Products

FSP, or
FDP

reticulo-endothelial
system
Kupffer's cells

When a fibrin clot dissolves, small pieces of fibrin are released. These pieces of fibrin are known as fibrin split products (FSP) or fibrin degradation products (FDP). Normally these pieces of fibrin are removed from the circulatory system by a network of cells known as the reticulo-endothelial system. The cells are found throughout the body, but are quite prevalent in the liver, where they are referred to as Kupffer's cells. The cells are phagocytic and remove the fibrin split products from the circulation. If the fibrin split products are not removed from the system, they become potent inhibitors of coagulation. FSP inhibits coagulation by preventing fibrin threads from cross-linking (forming the meshwork of a fibrin clot).

COAGULATION CASCADE / QUESTIONS

1. What is the end product of coagulation and what does it form?

2. For clots to form, protein binding must occur. What must be present for binding to occur?

3. What are the sources of phospholipids? Damaged tissue or activated platelets?

4. What would be the consequences if coagulation enzymes (serine proteases) circulated in the active form?

5. What is meant by the rate limiting step?

6. Explain the role of calcium in coagulation.

7. True or False. The coagulation cascade is like a chain reaction in which coagulation factors are activated to form a fibrin clot.

8. Name the two pathways involved in coagulation.

9. What phrase is another way to express pathway?

10. Under what conditions are the intrinsic and extrinsic activated?

11. True or False. Fibrin production is the result of either the intrinsic or the extrinsic pathway.

12. Explain the role of Vitamin K in blood coagulation.

13. What is Coumadin and how is it used?

14. Define clot lysis and its importance to blood flow.

15. What are the two pathways by which clot lysis occurs?

16. What does TPA mean?

17. What role does TPA play in the collection of postoperative shed blood?

18. How are fibrin split products (FSP) removed from the body?

19. If FSP were to remain in circulation, what would be the consequence?

20. Why are Kupffer's cells phagocytic and important in blood?

11 COAGULATION SYSTEM DISORDERS

All coagulation disorders cause bleeding to occur. Tests can be administered to determine the cause of bleeding. (For more details regarding the tests refer to the Appendix.) It is important to understand what can go wrong with the coagulation mechanism.

Disorders of Vascular Integrity

Vascular integrity is the normal state of vessels that allows blood to flow through in an uninterrupted fashion. It is the first component of hemostasis. Any time there is damage to the vessel, whether as a result of surgery or other cause, blood flow is interrupted and vascular integrity is lost.

The loss of vascular integrity can be divided into two categories: 1) surgical trauma or other trauma that interferes with blood flow, and 2) vessel abnormality due to artherosclerotic (cholesterol) plaque build-up on the vessel walls (fatty deposits). Genetic defects also can cause an abnormality in the structure of the vessel wall causing it to rupture at any time and without warning. Marfan's syndrome is a congenital defect that weakens vessel wall structure. The conditions described above can interfere with blood flow to the point that surgery is required to stop bleeding.

loss of vascular integrity

Coagulation Factor Disorders

When a coagulation factor is defective, bleeding occurs because fibrin stabilization of the platelet plug cannot take place. Disorders of the coagulation pathway are assessed by testing a sample of the patient's blood. (See Appendix for PT and PTT tests.)

There are many types of deficiencies of coagulation proteins. They are either congenital or acquired factor deficiencies. A congenital factor deficiency, such as

congenital factor deficiency

acquired factor
deficiency

hemophilia, involves a single protein abnormality, lasts for a person's lifetime, and is rare. Acquired factor deficiencies are different from the hereditary disorders in that they involve multiple factors, are nonhereditary, and are common. Examples are liver disease and renal failure. Usually, with an acquired factor deficiency a sudden onset of bleeding occurs.

Disseminated Intravascular Coagulation (DIC)

Disseminated intravascular coagulation is a condition that causes simultaneous widespread clotting and lysis in a diffuse uncontrolled manner throughout the body. Some types of injuries are more likely to give rise to DIC; for example, burns, crush injuries, vasculitis (inflammation of blood vessels), septicemia, viremia, and red cell hemolysis.

When a patient develops DIC the physician examines the steps in the coagulation process — vascular integrity, platelet formation, the coagulation cascade, and clot lysis — in order to determine the cause.

DIC and Vascular Integrity

While searching for the cause of DIC the physician first checks to see if loss of vascular integrity is responsible for the bleeding. When vascular integrity is lost, denuded endothelium presents itself and acts as a stimulus for the hemostatic process. When extensive surfaces are denuded of endothelium (as in the case of crush or burn injuries), large amounts of tissue phospholipids are released. As a result, platelet aggregation is activated and the coagulation cascade consumes large amounts of platelets and coagulation factors.

If vascular integrity is intact and not the cause of DIC, the physician next checks to determine whether abnormal platelet aggregation is the cause.

DIC and Platelet Aggregation

As previously indicated, platelet aggregation occurs when endothelial surfaces are exposed or tissue phospholipids are present. In abnormal conditions such as DIC, platelet aggregation occurs when large amounts of tissue phospholipids from damaged tissue are released. This causes aggregated platelets to release their own phospholipids, which stimulate and activate the clotting factors. When this happens, large amounts of platelets and clotting factors are used up by the body.

DIC and Consumption of Coagulation Factors

If the patient has suffered a crushing injury to the body, or a large area has been burned, or a malignant tumor is present, large amounts of phospholipids, especially tissue phospholipids, are exposed. In these cases, phospholipids cause widespread formation of fibrin (clotting) that leads to a consumption of the coagulation factors by the body. The labile (used once and destroyed) factors (V,VIII, and fibrinogen) are decreased. These factors are used only once in the coagulation process and are replenished by the liver. Other coagulation factors are used many times over and are not destroyed in the coagulation process.

DIC and Clot Lysis

When clotting (coagulation) takes place in the body, clot lysis also occurs, because the two events occur simultaneously. When clots are broken down, large amounts of fibrin split products (FSP) are released into the circulation. The more FSP that is present, the more normal clot formation is inhibited wherever needed in the body. If the concentration of FSP is high enough, platelets become dysfunctional.

The production and removal of FSP by the reticuloendothelial cells (Kupffer's cells) found in the liver determine the concentration of FSP in the circulation.

The Treatment of DIC

The treatment of DIC depends on the initial cause of the bleeding and whether consumption of the coagulation factors has occurred. However, until the cause of DIC is discovered, the consumed blood products (platelets, coagulation factors) must be replaced. If the bleeding is due to vascular integrity, cauterizing (stopping the bleeding by use of an electric current or suturing) may be all that is necessary to end DIC.

If the problem is not vascular integrity, then platelets or fresh frozen plasma (FFP) or cryoprecipitate must be administered to the patient (See p. 116.) They contain the components needed to help stop the bleeding. Remember that DIC consumes large amounts of these components and in order to stop the bleeding they must be replaced. Platelets are replaced by platelet transfusions. Factors V, VIII, and fibrinogen are replaced by transfusions of fresh frozen plasma, (FFP) or cryoprecipitate.

COAGULATION SYSTEM DISORDERS / QUESTIONS

1. True or false. Not all coagulation disorders cause bleeding to occur.

2. What is meant by vascular integrity?

3. When is vascular integrity lost?

4. Describe the two categories of the loss of vascular integrity.

5. Define hemostasis. Explain the function of platelets in hemostasis.

6. Why does bleeding occur when there are defective coagulation factors?

7. What is the difference between a congenital and an acquired coagulation deficiency?

8. Describe the two events in DIC.

9. What are two causes of DIC?

10. What event occurs when extensive surfaces are denuded of endothelium?

11. What is meant by the "consumption of the coagulation factors"?

12. In DIC what other event takes place in the body along with clotting?

13. When FSP is released in the circulation, clot formation is inhibited. If FSP concentration is high enough what happens to platelets?

12 PLATELET DISORDERS

platelet quality
platelet quantity

Platelets are the second component of hemostasis, the first being vascular integrity. Platelet disorders can involve both the quantity and quality of platelets. The quantity of platelets refers to the number of platelets in the circulation. If there are inadequate numbers of platelets, bleeding occurs because there are not enough platelets to form a plug over the damaged area. If the quality of the platelets is poor, bleeding also occurs due to poor platelet function.

The best way to determine whether platelet quantity or platelet quality is the problem is to compare two tests that are specific for platelets, the bleeding time and the platelet count. (See Appendix.)

A Low Platelet Count

A low platelet count has a number of causes, including bone tumors, radiation or chemotherapy, and the immune response to platelets by antibodies directed against platelets. The last can occur after multiple transfusions of platelets.

A significant cause of low platelet count can be the massive consumption (use by the clotting process) of platelets in platelet plug formation; for example, in conditions such as disseminated intravascular coagulation, often referred to as DIC. In DIC, platelets are used up by the body faster than they can be replaced. Platelet transfusion is the usual means of treating patients who are bleeding because of low platelet counts.

The Quality of Platelets

The quality of platelets can be affected by various drugs and conditions including the chemicals aspirin, protamine, and dextran; the presence of liver disease; the storage of platelets, which can affect their functional ability; and fibrin split products (FSP), which in high concentration can affect platelet function. Patients with poor platelet quality are treated by withholding drugs that affect platelet quality. Otherwise, patients may receive transfusions of platelets to improve platelet quality.

PLATELET DISORDERS / QUESTIONS

1.   Briefly describe two kinds of platelet disorders.

2.   Cite two causes of a low platelet count.

3.   What happens to platelets in DIC?

4.   Cite four drugs and/or conditions that can affect platelet quality.

13 BLOOD TRANSFUSION

An Introduction to Blood Transfusion

Blood transfusion is the infusion of blood or blood components into patients for treating a variety of surgical and medical conditions. Also called transfusion therapy, it involves one of the following: homologous (someone else's) blood, autologous (one's own) blood, or any blood component or substitutes. Because blood is a living tissue, a transfusion of whole blood or any of its components from one individual to another is considered a transplant, just like other tissue transplants (kidney, heart, liver, etc.). A blood transfusion may be indicated when blood is lost during trauma or surgery, to treat anemia and hemophilia, internal bleeding, and to replace a specific component destroyed by chemotherapy.

transfusion therapy
homologous blood
autologous blood

blood components

Before and after transfusion administration, several steps occur. For a transfusion, whole blood is collected from a donor or patient in a blood bag containing an anticoagulant/preservative. Blood is typed and cross matched for compatibility before administration to prevent transfusion reactions. Whole blood is usually processed into its components. Blood and blood components are tested for diseases and stored according to blood type and other criteria. They are then available for transfusion. During transfusion a patient must be monitored for a possible transfusion reaction.

Before the discovery of blood types in the early part of this century, blood transfusion was hazardous; it was successful only by chance. Over time the risks of disease transmission and transfusion reaction have been greatly reduced.

Blood Donation

The collection of blood or blood components from individuals for use in transfusions is called donation. Blood or its components for use in transfusion may be homologous (from volunteer donors) or autologous (from oneself). Any adult free of a serious disease or medical condition may donate blood. Certain conditions and diseases, however, prevent a person from donating. These include pregnancy, anemia (low RBC count), a previous history of malaria (a blood disease transmitted by the mosquito), a previous history of hepatitis (a disease affecting the liver), heart disease, and HIV infection (the AIDS virus). Adults may donate blood once every 3 or 4 months, because that is the time red blood cells need for regeneration.

Before a person can donate blood, he or she is given extensive medical questioning and a basic physical screening that includes temperature, pulse, blood pressure, and Hgb concentration. As long as the results of the medical screening are acceptable, donation begins.

Blood is usually withdrawn through veins in the crux of the elbow (forearm) (See Figure 36.). A tourniquet tightened around the upper arm causes the veins to

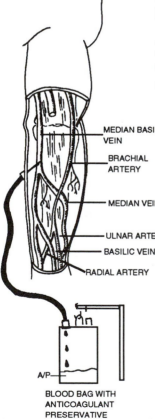

Figure 36 BLOOD DONATION

MEDIAN BASILIC VEIN

BRACHIAL ARTERY

MEDIAN VEIN

ULNAR ARTERY

BASILIC VEIN

RADIAL ARTERY

A/P

BLOOD BAG WITH ANTICOAGULANT PRESERVATIVE

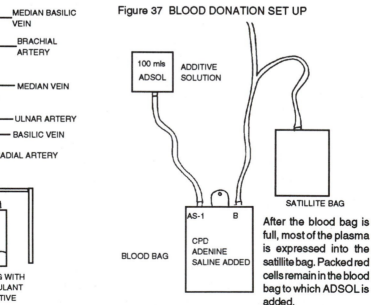

Figure 37 BLOOD DONATION SET UP

100 mls ADSOL

ADDITIVE SOLUTION

SATILLITE BAG

AS-1   B

CPD ADENINE SALINE ADDED

BLOOD BAG

After the blood bag is full, most of the plasma is expressed into the satillite bag. Packed red cells remain in the blood bag to which ADSOL is added.

bulge, making the insertion of a large bore needle easier. The needle is connected to a blood bag containing an anticoagulant/preservative, either CPD or CPDA-1, added to maintain RBC viability and prevent clotting. As blood slowly enters the bag, it mixes with the anticoagulant/preservative (See Figure 37.).

Approximately 1 pint of whole blood (500 ccs) is collected in a typical donation. This represents about 1/10 of the donor's total blood volume. It is called whole blood because it contains all the components of blood.

whole blood

After whole blood is collected, it is usually processed into its various components for storage and later use. The blood is tested for various viral markers for hepatitis, syphilis, and HIV. If the tests are negative, the blood components can be used for transfusions.

CPD and CPDA-1, the Citrate Anticoagulants/Preservatives

CPD and CPDA-1 are known collectively as the citrate anticoagulants/preservatives. They are commercially prepared solutions used only for the collection and storage of blood and blood components for transfusion. They are placed in blood bags by the manufacturer and have two functions: 1) to prevent collected blood from clotting, and 2) to provide nutrients for preserving and maintaining the viability of the red blood cells. If CPD and CPDA-1 were not used in collection, blood would clot within minutes. Either anticoagulant/ preservative can be used in the collection of whole blood, packed red cells, WBCs, platelets, and plasma.

red blood cell
viability

The solutions CPD and CPDA-1 contain the chemicals citrate, phosphate, and dextrose. CPDA-1 contains adenine. Citrate is the anticoagulant; the other chemicals are the preservatives.

citrate, phosphate,
dextrose

ATP

adenine

Citrate prevents clotting by binding the calcium (Ca^{++}) dissolved in the blood plasma and normally used in coagulation. Phosphate helps maintain high levels of adenosine triphosphate (ATP) in the blood. ATP is a high energy compound produced in the mitochondria (a cellular organelle). The mixture of glucose and O_2 in the cell produces ATP, which is a source of energy for most cellular reactions. High levels of ATP in RBCs allow better O_2 delivery to the tissues. Dextrose, also known as glucose, is a simple sugar that helps to maintain red blood cell viability. The chemical adenine in CPDA-1 aids the red blood cell in maintaining high levels of ATP. All the chemicals in the solutions, except citrate, aid in maintaining and extending the storage life of the red blood cell.

Whole blood collected in CPD can be refrigerated for 21 days, and that collected in CPDA-1 for 35 days. Whole blood and packed red cells are stored at 4 - 6^{0}C. Other cellular components require different storage temperatures.

ADSOL

additive solutions

After blood has been collected and the bag is full, most of the plasma is removed, either by spinning down (centrifuging) or by gravity. When plasma is removed from a unit of blood, packed red cells remain, along with a minimal amount of platelets, plasma, and WBCs. A clear solution called ADSOL is usually added to packed cells. ADSOL is the generic name for commercially prepared additive solutions that contain adenine, dextrose, saline, and mannitol. These chemicals aid in the preservation of red blood cells; they have no anticoagulative properties. The terms ADSOL and additive solutions may be used interchangeably.

About 100 mls of ADSOL are added to each bag or unit of packed red cells. Additive solutions must be added to packed cells within 72 hours of collection. ADSOL increases the storage shelf life of RBCs from the time of collection to 42 days by letting the cells carry on their normal metabolic processes. ADSOL can only be added to packed red blood cells. CPD is the anticoagulant used in whole blood collection when ADSOL is to be added.

Blood Storage

Blood is refrigerated in blood banks according to the ABO/Rh system. All units of blood are labeled by blood type: A+, B-, AB+, and so on. Platelets are also labeled this way. Banked blood is organized to ensure that blood and blood component transfusions are safely administered. Blood banks are operated by hospitals, the Red Cross, and private facilities.

ABO/Rh system

banked blood

Blood and blood components are banked (stored) according to standards established by the American Blood Bank Association. Each component is stored according to the time and temperature appropriate to maintain its viability. Blood and blood components are available from blood banks for patients as needs arise. For example, platelets are ready for patients actively bleeding due to thrombocytopenia or abnormal platelets, and plasma components are ready for hemophilia patients.

blood banks

Defects in Banked (Stored) Blood

The longer blood is stored the less viable its components are, a condition called storage lesion. Whole blood more than 24 hours old has few viable platelets or WBCs. There is also a decrease in the levels of clotting factors V and VIII, which, due to their short shelf life, are called labile factors. The other clotting factors maintain their levels of activity during storage and are called the stable factors.

storage lesion

labile factors

stable factors

Over time all stored units of blood suffer damage, a natural occurrence. Blood is a living tissue and must have a favorable environment to carry out cellular metabolism and maintain its viability.

89

Figure 38 CROSS MATCHING

I = Incompatible
C = Compatible

CROSS MATCHING

To determine blood compatibility for transfusion purposes, recipient serum (plasma minus fibrinogen) is mixed with the red cells of various donors. A donor's blood can be mixed with the recipient's blood in a transfusion if the cells do not clump.

RECIPIENT BLOOD GROUP

	O	A	B	AB
O	C	C	C	C
A	I	C	I	C
B	I	I	C	C
AB	I	I	I	C

DONOR BLOOD GROUP

Blood Typing and Cross Matching for Transfusions

Blood typing and cross matching must be done before transfusions can be performed. Blood typing determines blood type (A, B, AB, O); cross matching determines blood type compatibility between donor and recepient.(See Figure 38.)

blood type compatibility

By doing forward and reverse typing it is possible to determine a specific blood type through a process of elimination. Forward, or cell, typing determines the presence or absence of antigens A and B on red cell membranes. In reverse, or serum, typing the antibodies in serum can be determined through the use of reagents A and B, which are commercially prepared red cells. The Rh antigen on the red cell is determined in the same way and at the same time.

forward, or cell, typing

reverse, or serum, typing

reagents A and B

In cross matching, each donor's RBCs are tested with serum from the recipient to determine if the recipient has antibodies that can hemolyze (cause to burst) the donor's RBCs. When RBCs clump on the microscope slide the donor's blood should not be used in transfusion for the intended recipient. Absence of clumping indicates that the blood is compatible.

hemolyze

90

Blood Filtering

All blood products, except commercially prepared ones, should be transfused through a blood filter before administration to the patient. Blood filters filter out particulate matter such as hemolyzed red cells, cell fragments, plastic debris, and blood clots that may have formed during collection or storage. Other filters remove blood cells, specifically the white blood cells and platelets.

blood filters

Filters are available in many sizes and shapes. Standard blood filters have a pore size of about 150-270μ. Before or during transfusion filters trap unwanted debris that have formed in the blood after days of storage. Microaggregate (tiny) filters have a much smaller pore size (20-40μ). They trap microaggregate particles such as pieces of fibrin, fragments of platelets, and WBCs. Filters are placed in the IV line between the bag and the patient.

standard blood filters

microaggregate filters

Filters that remove white blood cells from blood and blood components are called leukocyte depletion filters. Units of packed RBCs and platelets contain small amounts of WBCs. These must be removed before transfusion to certain patients, who, as a result of multiple transfusions, react to the HLA (Human Leukocyte Antigens) on the membrane of the WBC. The antigen cannot be removed from the membrane; the WBC must be filtered out. The unit of blood may be filtered either before storage or at the bedside. It is preferable to remove WBCs before storage when they are intact. During storage many of them become fragmented, making removal more difficult.

leukocyte depletion

HLA

Blood Administration

Before a transfusion can begin, medical personnel must confirm that the blood registration numbers on the blood bag match blood bag numbers on the patient's chart. The right blood must be given to the right patient.

Y transfusion set

In preparation for transfusion a needle attached to a Y transfusion set is placed in the vein. A Y (double spike) transfusion set is most often used. (See Figures 39 and 40.) This set comes with a 170μ blood filter in place. The Y allows the blood unit and saline IV to be infused at the same time. The roller clamp on the IV line is opened and the blood or blood product and saline run into the patient. The IV line, a clear plastic tube, extends from the blood bag to the needle in the vein.

saline

An IV of normal saline (a salty solution) is attached to the IV line and infused along with the blood. Saline helps reduce the viscosity of blood and blood products so that they flow more freely. Saline is always the IV solution of choice when transfusing blood or blood components. It does not damage the cells as do other IV solutions, such as dextrose (causes hemolysis), Lactated Ringer's (increases Ca^{++}; blood may clot), or others.

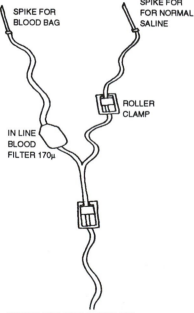

Figure 39 BLOOD ADMINISTRATION SET

SPIKE FOR BLOOD BAG

SPIKE FOR FOR NORMAL SALINE

ROLLER CLAMP

IN LINE BLOOD FILTER 170μ

NEEDLE ATTACHES AT THIS END

Medication is never added to a blood bag. All blood and blood components should be filtered before transfusion. During transfusion the patient's vital signs (pulse, blood pressure, temperature) are taken regularly for any possible sign of a transfusion reaction.

Figure 40 BLOOD TRANSFUSION

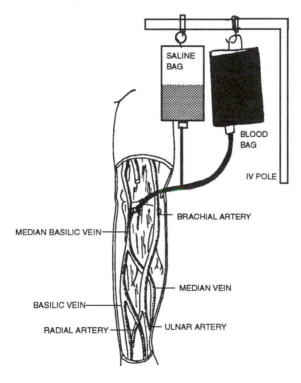

BLOOD TRANSFUSION / QUESTIONS

1. Define blood transfusion and two situations in which it may be required.

2. What is the difference between autologous and homologous blood?

3. Cite three persons who may not donate blood.

4. To donate blood the donor's Hgb concentration must be at a certain level. What is the level?

5. Why are CPD and CPDA-1 contained in blood bags? What is the term used to refer to both of them?

6. What is citrate and its function in CPD and CPDA-1?

7. Name the chemicals in CPD and CPDA-1.

8. CPDA-1 contains adenine. What role does this chemical have in maintaining red blood cell viability?

9. What is the storage life of whole blood and packed red cells collected in CPD? In CPDA-1?

10. When is ADSOL added to packed cells?

11. True or false. ADSOL may be added to WBCs and packed RBCs.

12. How much ADSOL is added to packed RBCs?

13. Blood banks store blood and platelets according to the ABO/ Rh system. Give two examples of how a unit of blood might be labeled.

14. Describe what happens to blood the longer it is stored.

15. Why must blood typing and cross matching be done before a transfusion can be administered?

16. In cross matching tests which is determined, blood type or compatibility?

17. True or false. Type AB blood can receive other blood types but cannot donate to another blood type.

18. All noncommercial blood products should be filtered before a transfusion. Cite three examples of particulate matter that filters trap.

19. What is the name of the filter that traps WBCs, and why must this filter must be used?

20. Give two reasons why saline is administered along with blood in a transfusion?

14 TRANSFUSION REACTIONS

There are many different kinds of transfusion reactions, such as hemolytic, febrile (nonhemolytic), and allergic. (See Chart 4.) They vary in severity and number of presenting symptoms. They can occur as a result of an incompatible ABO/Rh transfusion or sensitization to transfused WBCs, platelets, or plasma proteins.

When donor and recipient blood types are incompatible, a transfusion reaction occurs. In a transfusion reaction, antigens on the red blood cell membrane (A, B, or Rh) of the donor react to, or are incompatible with, the antibodies (anti-A, anti-B, or Rh antibodies) in the recipient's plasma. In a transfusion reaction blood group antibodies in the recipient's plasma cause the donor red cells to hemolyze (burst).(See Figure 41.) Because Type O blood has no antigens on the RBC, there is usually no problem in a transfusion.

An immediate life-threatening situation can develop in an incompatible ABO blood transfusion. An anaphylactic shock-like condition, which can be fatal, can be observed in the patient.

ABO/Rh transfusion

recepient's plasma

donor red cells

Figure 41 RED CELL LYSIS DUE TO A TRANSFUSION REACTION

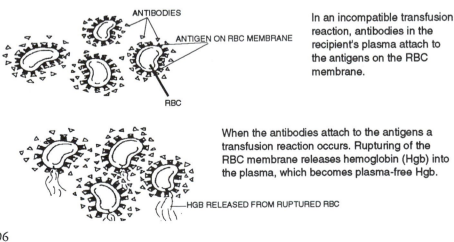

ANTIBODIES

ANTIGEN ON RBC MEMBRANE

RBC

In an incompatible transfusion reaction, antibodies in the recipient's plasma attach to the antigens on the RBC membrane.

When the antibodies attach to the antigens a transfusion reaction occurs. Rupturing of the RBC membrane releases hemoglobin (Hgb) into the plasma, which becomes plasma-free Hgb.

HGB RELEASED FROM RUPTURED RBC

96

Any transfusion reaction can include some or all of the following symptoms: reddening of the face (flushing), increased rate of breathing (hyperventilation), increased heart rate (tachycardia), sense of fright, patchy blotches of skin (urticaria), shortness of breath (dyspnea), chest pressure, and back pain. A feeling of nausea may occur and, in some instances, progress to vomiting. Cyanosis (bluish color to skin) and fever in the range of 102-105° F may be evident. Severe back pain in a transfusion reaction is caused by remnants of the red cell membranes blocking the microvasculature (capillaries) of the kidneys, which can cause renal failure.

Renal Failure

The most feared ABO transfusion reaction is renal failure, the delayed complication caused by hemolysis. This event can be triggered even when only a small amount of incompatible ABO blood is administered. Renal shutdown can occur, and when it does the patient is slowly poisoned because the kidneys cannot remove impurities from the blood. When the kidneys no longer work, dialysis usually is required to cleanse the blood. Dialysis is done 2 or 3 times a week or until kidney function returns to normal.

When large amounts of ABO-incompatible blood are given, there is almost always some renal tubular necrosis (damage to the tubules in the kidney). In certain patients, this condition is irreversible and damage to the kidney is permanent. Another reason it is essential to type and cross match donor RBCs and recipient serum.

Chart 1: Common Signs and Symptoms of a Transfusion Reaction

Signs and symptoms:

- Fever and chills
- Chest and back pain
- Sore aching muscles
- Headache
- Numbness and tingling
- Pain at infusion site
  (needle puncture site)
- Wheezing and coughing
- Dyspnea (shortness of breath)
- Tachypnea (increased rate of breathing)
- Stomach cramps and diarrhea
- Nausea and vomiting
- Increase or decrease of blood pressure
- Irregular heartbeat
- Flushing of the skin (reddening)
- Cyanosis (blue coloring)
- Edema (swelling)
- Changes in amount of urine;
  either increase or decrease
- Dark color to urine
- Renal failure
- Bleeding
- Urticaria (rash and hives)
- Sweating

Chart 2: Steps to Follow When Signs and Symptoms of a Transfusion Reaction Occur

- Stop the transfusion immediately
- Maintain IV of 0.9% normal saline to maintain venous access for drug administration
- Report incident to physician and blood bank
- Check blood bag tags and numbers with those in the patient chart
- Treat symptoms appropriately
- Send unused portion of blood in blood bag and the administration set to the blood bank
- Collect and send blood and urine samples to the lab
- Document the transfusion reaction and treatment thoroughly

Chart 3: Transfusion Reaction in the Unconscious or Anesthetized Patient

Signs and symptoms:	*Actions:*
• Weak or absent pulse • Decrease in blood pressure • Small amount of urine; possibly none produced • Fever • Increase or decrease in the heart rate • Increase in amount of bleeding during surgery • Visible signs of Hgb in the urine (hemoglobinuria)	Stop the transfusion immediately and monitor the patient closely. Initiate treatment.

Chart 4: Acute Transfusion Reactions

Acute Hemolytic
Description: A serious life-threatening reaction
Causes: Transfusion of ABO incompatible blood, packed cells, or components. Antibodies in recipient plasma attach to the transfused red blood cells, leading to lysis of the transfused red blood cells.
Signs and Symptoms: See Chart 1. Patients can experience many of the serious complications such as renal failure, anaphalactic shock, pulmonary edema, etc.
Actions: Stop the transfusion immediately. The patient should be monitored closely.

Anaphylactic Shock
Description: The most severe transfusion reaction
Causes: Transfusion of IgA proteins from a donor into a recipient who is IgA deficient. The recipient has developed antibodies to the IgA protein.
Signs and Symptoms: See Chart 1. Includes the most serious signs and symptoms, e.g., shock, cyanosis, kidney failure, etc.
Actions: This is a full-blown medical emergency and must be attended to immediately.

Circulatory Overload
Description: Signs similar to congestive heart failure or pulmonary edema
Causes: Transfusion of fluid into patient faster than his or her circulatory system can accommodate.
Signs and Symptoms: Mostly pulmonary
Actions: Eliminate excess fluid from the body with diuretics

continued

Chart 4 *contin.*

Mild allergic
Description: Usually a relatively mild reaction
Causes: Sensitization to foreign plasma proteins of the donor
Signs and Symptoms: See Chart 2. Patients can experience some of the milder transfusion reactions, e.g., uticaria, headache, dizziness, etc. Rarely progresses to more serious complications.
Actions: Patient should be watched for other more serious complications.

Sepsis
Description: Usually not a problem depending on bacterial contaminant
Causes: Transfusion of contaminated blood or blood components
Signs and Symptoms: See Chart 1. Patients can experience high fever, chills, diarrhea, vomiting, hypotension, and shock.
Actions: Blood cultures should be taken from the recipient and appropriate antibiotics administered. Patient should be monitored closely.

Febrile, nonhemolytic
Description: The most common reaction following a blood transfusion
Causes: Sensitization to antigens on the white blood cells, platelets, or plasma proteins of the donor
Signs and Symptoms: See Chart 1. Patients can experience nonlife-threatening signs and symptoms such as fever, headache, chills, etc. Rarely progresses to more serious complications.
Actions: Treat symptoms as necessary

TRANSFUSION REACTION / QUESTIONS

1. Explain what happens as the result of an incompatible transfusion reaction.

2. True or false, Type O blood has antigens on the RBC membrane, which can result in a transfusion reaction.

3. What is released from a ruptured RBC in a transfusion reaction?

4. Describe five signs and symptoms of a transfusion reaction.

5. Renal failure is a severe transfusion reaction and can lead to patient death. Explain why.

6. What is the first step in dealing with a transfusion reaction?

15 TRANSFUSION AND DISEASE TRANSMISSION

For hundreds of years homologous blood has been used successfully – and unsuccessfully – in blood and blood component replacement therapy. Transfusions save many lives, but reactions and disease transmission via transfusion can result in serious complications and even death to recipients.

Blood should be screened before transfusion for transmittible bacterial and viral diseases. These include hepatitis B and C, viruses that affect the liver in varying degrees of severity; HTLV-I, a precursor of leukemia; HIV; and the disease syphilis, a sexually transmitted bacterium. If a test result for any of the above diseases is positive, the blood is discarded.

During the 1980s the fear of contracting AIDS forced the public and medical community to question the safety of homologous blood and blood products. Closer scrutiny and testing of donors have greatly reduced the incidence of disease transmission via transfusion.

AIDS

Any potential blood donor must have his or her blood tested for antibodies in the plasma developed against the Human Immunodeficiency Virus, or HIV, the virus that causes AIDS. The enzyme-linked immunoassay test (ELISA) is used to determine whether the body has developed antibodies to HIV. The ELISA test is not foolproof; there is no guarantee that blood tested for antibodies to HIV is not contaminated with the virus. The ELISA test measures the antibodies produced by the body in response to HIV infection and not the presence of the virus itself. An individual who wants to confirm HIV negativity should be retested in six months. Any time the ELISA test is positive for HIV the blood is further tested by the Western blot, a more involved confirmatory test.

HIV

ELISA

103

Figure 42 THE AIDS VIRUS

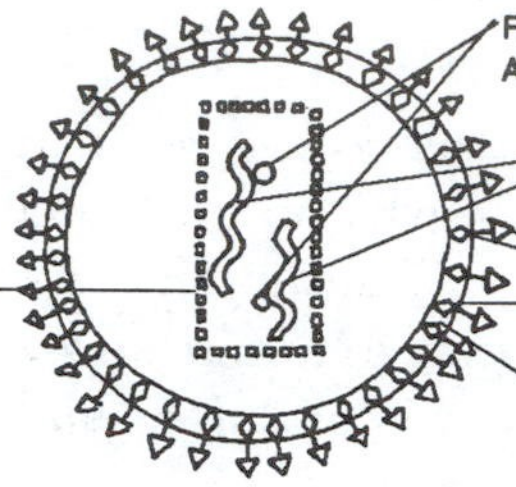

REVERSE TRANSCRIPTASE (ENZYMES THAT ALLOW THE VIRUS TO CONVERT RNA TO DNA)

IDENTICAL STRANDS OF RNA

CORE POLYPEPTIDES

PROTEINS
VIRAL ENVELOPE
PHOSPHOLIPID BILAYER

The production of antibodies in response to an infection is not immediate. It takes time for the body to build up an antibody level that registers a positive test result. Therefore, a recently infected individual may be HIV positive, but not have sufficient levels of antibody to test positive. He or she tests negative for HIV and as a donor can transmit the virus. An HIV positive individual can be symptom-free of AIDS for a period of time, depending on the individual. He or she may have minor to severe infections in a stage referred to as AIDS-related complex, or ARC. Some individuals are not strong enough to survive this stage.

ARC

HIV is transmitted in a number of ways. There is a small but serious risk associated with contaminated blood transfusions. Other forms of HIV transmission include IV drug use (sharing contaminated needles), sexual, or by the exchange of body fluids (sperm, vaginal secretions, breast milk, urine, bowel contents, and menstrual blood).

retroviruses

RNA

DNA

HIV belongs to the family of viruses called retroviruses. (The AIDS virus is so small that a billion can be put on the head of a pin.) All retroviruses have RNA (ribonucleic acid) as their genetic material, chemicals that make up the genes of an organism. Most living organisms, including humans, have DNA (deoxyribonucleic acid) as their genetic material. Retroviruses come equipped with special chemicals (enzymes) that enable them to convert their RNA into DNA and insert this newly formed DNA into the DNA of the host cell. Viral DNA takes control of the host cell's DNA and replicates the virus within the cell. The host cell then becomes a factory for producing viruses.

Retroviruses are slow growing, which means that a person can be infected for a long time before the signs and symptoms of AIDS become evident. The symptoms of full-blown AIDS are infections and tumors such as Karposi's sarcoma, *Pneumocystis carinii* pneumonia, thrush (a fungal infection), etc. When any of these symptoms develop in an HIV positive patient, he or she is considered to have AIDS.

The infections associated with AIDS are called opportunistic infections, because they appear in individuals with severely weakened immune systems and not in those with healthy immune systems. People can live with AIDS for years. In most cases, however, the body succumbs to the opportunistic infections and dies.

opportunistic infections

The Role of T-4 Lymphocytes and Macrophages in AIDS

AIDS patients lack some of the major players of the immune system, namely, the T-4 lymphocytes (a subset of T cells) and macrophages. These are the two cell types HIV attacks and destroys. Without them, the body cannot conquer any disease.

T-4 lymphocytes and macrophages have communication lines in the immune response. Macrophages eat foreign antigenic particles (bacteria and viruses) and digest them (break into small pieces). After digestion, the macrophage exposes antigenic particles on the outside of its cellular surface and presents them to the T-4 lymphocytes. These cells decode the information in the particles and use it to direct the B-lymphocytes to change into plasma cells. The plasma cells produce the specific antibodies that respond to the foreign antigens.

In AIDS patients, cell communication lines in the immune response are destroyed by HIV. Recognition of foreign organisms does not occur, and therefore no antibody production takes place.

105

TRANSFUSION AND DISEASE TRANSMISSION / QUESTIONS

1. Why should blood be tested prior to a transfusion?

2. Name three diseases that can be transmitted by a transfusion.

3. True or false. ELISA is the single best test to determine whether a donor has HIV, because it determines the presence of the AIDS virus.

4. True or false. HIV cannot be transmitted by blood transfusion.

5. What happens after the AIDS virus converts its RNA into DNA and then inserts its DNA into the host cell's DNA?

6. What is the name for the kind of virus that causes AIDS?

7. Explain the significance of opportunistic infections to the AIDS patient. Give two examples of an opportunistic infection.

8. At what point is an HIV positive person considered to have AIDS?

9. Explain the meaning of the following as it relates to AIDS patients: Recognition of foreign organisms does not occur, and therefore no antibody production takes place.

16 METHODS OF AUTOLOGOUS BLOOD RECOVERY

Autologous Blood

Autologous blood is the best possible blood for an individual to receive, because there is no chance of disease transmission or a transfusion reaction. The reinfusion of one's own blood is called autotransfusion. Autologous blood recovery is the collection of the patient's own blood or blood components for transfusion. Using autologous blood decreases the demand for homologous blood.

Currently, there are three autologous blood recovery methods by which patients may receive their own blood during or after surgery: 1) predonation, 2) intraoperative blood salvage, and 3) postoperative (wound drainage) collection.

Predonation

Predonation is an autologous method used for scheduled surgical procedures in which the surgeon expects significant blood loss. The operations include cardiac, vascular, liver, and orthopedic, among others. To predonate blood the surgical patient must have a Hgb concentration of 11 g/dl and a Hct of 33%. If the Hgb concentration and the Hct are lower, predonation is not recommended. A low reading indicates anemia and donation would cause the donor to become more anemic.

Each week for a few weeks before surgery the patient donates a pint of his or her own blood. By the time of surgery the patient may have as many as four units of autologous blood in reserve in case a blood transfusion is required during the operation. If the autologous blood is not used, it may be used to transfuse another individual, but only if it passes the mandatory tests required for homologous blood.

Intraoperative Blood Salvage

Intraoperative blood salvage is the collection and reinfusion of blood shed by the patient during surgery. This method of autologous blood recovery involves the use of two types of special equipment: 1) wash devices that collect and wash (cleanse) blood before reinfusion and 2) nonwash devices that collect and reinfuse blood to the patient without washing it. The wash system is also referred to as a cell processor. The nonwash device includes a sterile suction cannister that collects the blood shed during surgery. The blood collected by these devices is mixed with anticoagulants (nonwash, CPD; wash, heparin).

The wash and nonwash devices are used for different surgical procedures. Neither can be used for every surgical procedure. Intraoperative salvage is not recommended during open bowel (intestinal), bladder, and cancer surgeries or when the patient is septic (has an infection). Reinfused blood in these cases would expose the patient to possibly dangerous contaminants.

The wash devices eliminate the following from autologous blood: heparin (an anticoagulant), plasma-free Hgb, hemolyzed red cell membranes, drugs and other solutions used during surgery, surgical debris, and other contaminates. All of these may cause complications for the patient. During surgery a wash device collects blood in a spinning centrifuge bowl located within the cell processor. When the bowl is full the device washes the blood with 1000 ccs of normal saline. Washed blood lacks clotting factors, platelets, plasma, and WBCs. These components are washed away into a waste bag. The patient is reinfused only with RBCs and a small amount of saline.

Wash devices are used in cardiac, liver transplant, orthopedic, vascular, and other surgeries. They are used exclusively in cardiac, liver, and orthopedic surgeries due to the amount of debris generated, drugs used, and, in some cases, the quantity of blood shed.

wash devices

nonwash devices

The nonwash devices do not remove surgical debris, except particulates that are trapped by the blood filter inserted in the IV line. Autologous blood reinfused by a nonwash device may contain plasma-free Hgb, debris generated during surgery, and active tissue factors. Nonwash devices are not designed to keep up with the rapid blood loss that can occur in cardiac and liver surgery.

The decision to wash or not to wash blood is a matter of personal preference by the surgeon. Some surgeons believe that unwashed blood presents no problems to the patient.

Postoperative Wound Drainage

Wound drainage refers to the collection and reinfusion of blood shed postoperatively. The procedure, which has become popular recently, is a method of autologous blood recovery that helps reduce the use of homologous blood in transfusions given after surgery. In some surgeries, particularly total hip and knee replacements and the correction of spinal deformities, blood is likely to be shed postoperatively. Wound drainage devices collect and reinfuse this blood, which in the past would have been discarded and replaced by homologous blood. Wound drainage collection systems are smaller versions of the devices used to collect and reinfuse blood intraoperatively.

METHODS OF AUTOLOGOUS BLOOD RECOVERY / QUESTIONS

1. Why is autologous blood preferred to homologous blood in a transfusion?

2. What are the three methods of autologous blood recovery?

3. Name three operations for which a surgeon would required predonation and the reason why.

4. True or false. An Hgb concentration of 11 g/dl and a Hct of 33% would prevent a person from predonating his or her blood.

5. Explain the term intraoperative blood salvage.

6. List the two kinds of equipment used in intraoperative blood salvage, explaining the chief difference between them.

7. Cite five contaminates that wash devices eliminate from autologous blood.

8. When washed blood is reinfused what components are washed away? Reinfused?

9. True or false. The decision to use a wash or nonwash device is a matter of personal preference by the surgeon.

10. How does postoperative wound drainage reduce the use of homologous blood in transfusion after surgery?

17 COMPONENT THERAPY

Component therapy refers to the use of a specific blood component to treat certain conditions or diseases such as anemia, leukemia, thrombocytopenia, and hemophilia. Blood component therapy has radically changed the way blood and blood products are used. In the early days of transfusion medicine, whole blood was given to patients who needed blood for any reason. Today, whole blood is rarely administered to a patient and then only when blood loss is significant.

In component therapy, whole blood is collected and processed into its various components (RBCs, WBCs, platelets, and plasma), which then become available for treating many patients. For example, anemic patients (those with a low RBC count) need only RBCs, not whole blood. Because they are often normovolemic (have normal circulating blood volume), a unit of whole blood overloads their vascular system, a condition referred to as circulatory overload. An increase in blood volume can have serious consequences for the patient. A transfusion of packed RBCs properly treats their condition. Aside from being unhealthy, transfusing a unit of whole blood when it is not needed is wasteful.

whole blood

Some blood components are prepared by blood banks while others are prepared by pharmaceutical companies as purified concentrations of plasma proteins. The latter include coagulation factor concentrates, albumin and plasma protein fraction, immune serum globulin, and erythropoietin.

purified concentrations
of plasma proteins

Whole Blood

A unit of whole blood is comprised of RBCs, WBCs, platelets, and plasma, with a volume of 450 mls. A unit of whole blood also has 63 mls of anticoagulant/preservative (CPD or CPDA-1) added to it. The Hct of whole blood is usually between 36-44%.

transfusion
components

Today, whole blood is rarely used in transfusion. It is usually processed into its components. If, however, a patient has massive blood loss, usually greater than 25% of the total blood volume, a unit of whole blood may be used. No components are removed from whole blood to be used in transfusion. An infusion of whole blood improves the patient's ability to transport O_2 (RBCs). It also increases the circulating blood volume (plasma). The infusion of a unit of whole blood raises the Hct (number of RBCs) of a patient by about 3%. Because it raises the Hgb concentration by about 1 g/dl, whole blood increases the ability of the patient to transport O_2.

Apheresis

cytapheresis
hemapheresis
plasmapheresis
plateletpheresis

single-donor apheresis

Apheresis is the removal of a specific blood component or components from the circulation of a patient or donor. (Apheresis means separation.) The removal of RBCs and WBCs is referred to as cytapheresis or hemapheresis, plasma removal as plasmapheresis, and platelet removal as plateletpheresis. When there is only one donor, apheresis is called single-donor apheresis. When there are multiple donors, the process is referred to as apheresis. Single-donor apheresis is better for the patient because the risks of a transfusion reaction and disease transmission are reduced.

A specific blood component from a donor may be used to treat a disease or medical condition. For example, HLA-matched platelets are given to people who have received multiple transfusions and have built up numerous antibodies to different platelets, i.e., they are sensitized to HLA and matched platelets reduce the possibility of a reaction.

therapeutic apheresis

In therapeutic apheresis a specific problematic component is removed from the patient's blood and, depending on the condition, may or may not be replaced with an equivalent donor component. For example, in sickle-cell disease as many abnormal RBCs as possible are removed from the patient's circulation and replaced with homologous packed cells. In this disease the RBC Hgb molecule changes shape after it releases O_2 to the tissues. As a result, the cells take on a sickle shape and block the microvasculature of many organs. Transfused homologous packed cells have normal Hgb and do not sickle. In the disease polycythemia there are too many RBCs, which increase blood viscosity. The result is circulatory blockage similar to that in sickle-cell disease. Patients with polychthemia may have RBCs removed to reduce viscosity; RBCs are not replaced, just withdrawn.

In apheresis, blood is collected and spun in a bowl by an automated machine called a cell separator. Sterile disposable tubing sets in the cell separator collect the component. IV lines from the tubing set are inserted into one or two veins of the donor or patient. Blood is drawn into the bowl and spun by centrifuging (high speed spinning), which separates the component from the blood for collection. The speed of the centrifuge bowl can be adjusted to isolate a specific component. Blood components that are not needed are reinfused back to the donor via the IV line connecting the bowl to the individual.

cell separator

centrifuging

The apheresis procedure must be done 6 - 8 times per session to collect the desired amount of blood. There are two reasons for this: the small size of the separator bowl and the need to maintain donor blood volume. The blood balance of the donor is virtually unaffected because so little of the component is removed.

Packed Red Cells

Packed cells are used for patients losing blood during surgery, for patients with different kinds of anemia, and other conditions such as leukemia.

A unit of packed RBCs is prepared from a unit of whole blood. Plasma, 200-250 mls, is removed from the unit. ADSOL, 100 mls, is added to the packed red cells to keep them metabolically active. Packed RBCs

ADSOL

plasma

simply means that most of the plasma has been removed from the unit of blood. Removing plasma increases the concentration of RBCs, which in turn raises the Hct of the packed RBCs in the unit. Plasma removed from whole blood can be broken down into other components, including fresh frozen plasma (FFP), cryoprecipitate, and albumin, etc.

CPD or CPDA-1

Packed RBCs are collected in an anticoagulant/ preservative, either CPD or CPDA-1. Packed RBCs collected in CPD have a shelf life of 21 days and a Hct of 38-40%. Blood collected in CPDA-1 has a shelf life of 35 days and a Hct of 70-80%. Packed RBCs collected in additive solutions (ADSOL) have a shelf life of 42 days and a Hct of 55-60%. The lower Hct is due to the volume of ADSOL that has been added. The shelf life of packed cells varies depending on whether they have been supplied with an additive solution. Additive solutions can be added only to packed RBCs and to no other blood component. Packed red cells are stored at 4-6°C.

Packed red cells should be ABO/Rh compatible, but in some emergency situations this requirement may be disregarded and O- cells administered. Packed cells should not be transfused for volume expansion or to improve wound healing.

Leukocyte Poor (Depleted) Red Blood Cells

HLA antigens

leukocyte depletion

Patients who receive multiple transfusions are exposed to many antigens. They are sensitive to HLA antigens on the WBC membrane. To prevent sensitization to HLA, the WBCs are removed in a process called leukocyte depletion. Leukocyte depletion is accomplished by irradiation (by gamma rays), washing, centrifuging (high speed spinning), washing of frozen RBCs, or filtering through a microaggregate filter.

White Blood Cells

114

White blood cells, specifically granulocytes, usually are

prepared for transfusion by single-donor apheresis. single-donor apheresis
They are used to transfuse the following patients: those
who lack the ability to fight off infections (weakened
immune system), those with decreased neutrophils
(neutropenia), and those who do not respond to
antibiotics. These patients often are undergoing
chemotherapy for leukemia (cancer of the WBCs) or
bone marrow replacement therapy. Sepsis (infections)
can occur in both cases.

Today, WBCs are used in transfusion infrequently,
partly because powerful antibiotics are available. WBCs
are stored at room temperature, 20-24°C and have a
shelf life of 24 hours. They should be ABO/Rh
compatible.

Platelets

Platelets are used to treat bleeding disorders due to a
low platelet count (thrombocytopenia), abnormal
platelets, or destruction of platelets as in DIC. Platelets
for use in transfusion are prepared from individual
units of whole blood by centrifugation. Platelets are
collected during centrifuging, with only a small amount
of plasma trapped in the process. The number of
platelets in a unit is 5×10^{10}, suspended in 50-70 ml of
plasma.

Platelets should be Rh compatible with the recipient,
but they do not have to be ABO compatible. They are
stored at 20-24°C, which is about 18 degrees warmer
than the temperature at which blood is stored. At
colder temperatures, platelets become inactive and
useless. Platelets have a shelf life of 5 days, which
means they must be used within that time.

When a large volume of platelets is needed, as in heart
surgery, liver surgery, and DIC, platelets from multiple
donors often are administered. Called pooled platelets, pooled platelets
they are pooled for patients who have very low platelet
counts and need a large transfusion. Pooled platelets,
however, increase patient exposure to transmittable

115

diseases and to the formation of platelet antibodies by the patient.

Platelets usually are not successful in stopping bleeding caused by excessive platelet destruction as in ITP (idiopathic thrombocytopenia), untreated DIC, septicemia (infection), or hypersplenism (in which the spleen destroys too many blood cells). A platelet transfusion does not stop bleeding because platelets are destroyed faster than they can be replaced.

During or after platelet transfusion it is not uncommon for patients to have fever and chills. If a transfusion reaction does occur, the transfusion should be stopped immediately. Aspirin should not be adminstered to treat the fever because it inhibits platelet function.

plateletpheresis

HLA

Platelets are collected from a single donor in a process called plateletpheresis. The volume of platelets collected is equivalent to 5 or 6 units of pooled platelets. Apheresis platelets are given to patients who have become sensitized to HLA and have developed platelet antibodies (antibodies against platelets).

Plasma Components

Plasma components are used for many conditions including bleeding disorders, liver disease, burns, shock, and massive blood loss.

Plasma that has been collected may be separated (processed) into its various components: cryoprecipitate, fresh frozen plasma, coagulation factor concentrates (factors VIII and IX), albumin, plasma protein factor, and immune serum globulin.

Fresh Frozen Plasma (FFP)

FFP is used to treat clotting factor deficiencies including multiple factor deficiency resulting from liver disease, DIC, and coagulation complications after bypass surgery. It should not be used for volume expansion.

Fresh frozen plasma is prepared from whole blood. As soon as possible after collection, plasma is separated from whole blood and quickly frozen. Plasma treated this way retains most of the activity of factors V and VIII. Plasma can be stored up to 1 year at -18°C. The volume of a unit of plasma is 200-250 mls.

factors V and VIII

Cryoprecipitate

Cryoprecipitate is a concentrated solution of coagulation proteins found in the plasma. It is produced by freezing freshly collected plasma. During freezing a white precipitate forms a layer on top of the frozen plasma. This "buffy coat" is the cryoprecipitate. To collect the cryoprecipitate, a unit of FFP is thawed and the white precipitate is removed. Cryoprecipitate contains high concentrations of factors VIII, XIII, and fibrinogen.

FFP

factors VIII, XIII, fibrinogen

Cryoprecipitate is used to treat hemophilia A, von Willebrand's disease, DIC, and congenital and acquired factor deficiencies, among others. "Cryo," as it is called, must be ABO compatible to prevent hemolysis of the recipient's blood.

Cryo

Coagulation Factor Concentrates

Coagulation factor concentrates are powdered (lyophilized) concentrates removed from units of pooled donor plasma. The concentrates contain large amounts of factors VIII and IX. Factor VIII concentrate is used to treat Hemophilia A. Factor IX concentrate is used to treat Hemophilia B, or Christmas disease, and other factor deficiencies. The concentrates are prepared by heating or washing with a detergent, and, therefore are unlikely to transmit viral diseases.

factors VIII and IX

Albumin and Plasma Protein Fraction (PPF)

Albumin is a naturally occurring blood protein that makes up part of the plasma. It is used to treat patients who have lost a large volume of blood, a condition called hypovolemia, and those with low blood protein levels. ABO testing is not required before giving an albumin transfusion. Albumin does not need to be given through a blood filter, because it does not contain clots or debris. Albumin does not transmit AIDS in transfusion because it is heated to 60° C for 10 hours during the component preparation process.

Plasma Protein Fraction, or PPF, is another protein component separated from plasma. It is less pure than albumin because it contains a higher percent of other plasma proteins. PPF does not transmit disease in transfusion because it is pasteurized (heated to kill organisms) in the process of preparation.

HDN

Albumin and PPF are used to treat patients with burns, massive bleeding, or liver failure. Such patients need volume expansion other than by crystalloids, which are deficient in proteins. Albumin and PPF also are used to treat hemolytic disease of the newborn, or HDN, a disease in which the presence of Rh antibodies in the mother hemolyze the Rh+ RBCs of the newborn.

Immune Serum Globulin

gamma globulin

passive immunization

hypogammaglobulinemia

Immune serum globulin, also known as IgG or gamma globulin, is a concentrated solution of antibodies prepared from plasma. Patients infected with an organism that is too powerful for their immune system to destroy may receive plasma from a donor who has been exposed to or had the same infection. Antibodies are removed from the donor plasma and transfused into the recipient to provide antibodies already formed against the antigen. This is called passive immunization, because the immunity comes from sources outside the body. Immune serum globulin is also given to patients who are deficient in gamma globulin, a condition called hypogammaglobulinemia.

Erythropoietin

Erythropoietin, a naturally occurring protein hormone produced and released by the kidney cells, stimulates stem cells to develop into RBCs. Erythropoietin is released from the kidney cells when blood passing through the kidneys is low in O_2. Patients with poor kidney function are anemic, because often they are unable to produce erythropoietin. Before its discovery, kidney patients were given a unit of packed RBCs to maintain a normal Hct level.

Synthetic erythropoietin is now produced by molecular technology. It is used for patients with kidney disease. A promising therapy, synthetic erythropoietin does in fact stimulate the stem cells to make RBCs. In addition, it causes few side effects for the patient.

synthetic erythropoietin

CHART 5: BLOOD COMPONENTS

PRODUCT	WHOLE BLOOD	PACKED RBCS	PACKED RED CELLS	PLATELETS	WBCS GRANULOCYTES	FRESH FROZEN PLASMA (FFP)
AC/P	CPD, CPDA-1	CPD, CPDA-1	ADSOL	CPD, CPDA-1	CPD, CPDA-1	CPD, CPDA-1
HCT OF PRODUCT	36-44%	80%	55-60%	—	—	—
VOLUME OF UNIT	500 mls	250 mls	300-350 mls	50-70 mls	200-400 mls with platelets;100-200 mls in unit if no platelets in units	—
DISEASE TRANSMISSION	Yes	Yes	Yes	Yes	Yes	Yes, except CMV
ABO/Rh COMPATIBILITY	ABO and Rh	ABO and Rh	ABO and Rh	Rh compatibility necessary; ABO compatibility preferred, not necessary	ABO and Rh	ABO
USES IN TREATMENT	Rarely used; may be used for massive blood loss or severe burns	RBC replacement; often used with crystalloids to increase Hct and volume	RBC replacement; often used with crystalloids to increase Hct and volume	To increase platelet count	For individuals with low WBC count or unresponsive to antibiotics	To increase clotting factor levels; valuable in treating factor deficiencies when concentrates not available
INCIDENTALS	Rh- blood may be given to Rh+ individuals; presence of WBCs and platelets may cause sensitization; should be filtered. Storage: 21 days in CPD, 35 in CPDA-1	2 times the Hct of unit of whole blood; should be filtered. Storage: 21 days in CPD, 35 in CPDA-1	ADSOL increases storage time to 42 days; should be filtered	Rh- patients may need Rh+ platelets and possibly RhoGAM. Multiple platelet transfusions may sensitize patients to HLA antigens, requiring HLA-matched platelets. Blood filter (170μ). Storage: 20-24°C Shelf life: 5 days	Not accepted by Food and Drug Administration (FDA). HLA problems possible with transfusions. Storage: 20-24°C. Shelf life: 24 hrs	Often used after bypass surgery. Storage: -18°C Shelf life: 1 yr

CHART 5: BLOOD COMPONENTS *contin.*

PRODUCT	CRYOPRE-CIPITATE	COAGULATION FACTOR CONCEN-TRATE; FACTOR VIII	FACTOR IX	COLLOID SOLUTIONS ALBUMIN	PLASMA PROTEIN FRACTION (PPF)	IMMUNE SERUM GLOBULIN
AC/p	—	—	—	—	—	—
HCT OF PRODUCT	—	—	—	—	—	—
VOLUME OF UNIT	10-20 mls	Amount of FVIII in mgs varies by manufacturer	Amount of FIX in mgs varies by manufacturer	200 and 500 mls 5%; 50 and 100 mls 25%	5% solution of albumin in saline; 200-500 mls	Varies by manufacturer
DISEASE TRANSMISSION	Yes	No; reduced risk	No; reduced risk	No	No	Yes, some, but not AIDS
ABO/Rh COMPATIBILITY	Preferred, but not necessary	Plasma compatible, but not necessary	Plasma compatible, but not necessary	No	No	—
USES IN TREATMENT	To increase levels of factors VIII, XIII, fibrinogen, and von Willebrand's factor	For treatment of FVIII deficiency (Hemophilia A)	Hemophilia B (Christmas disease)	Volume expansion when crystalloids inadequate (shocks, burns, liver failure, hemorrhage); used in severe liver disease	Initial treatment of hemorrhagic shock caused by burns; used in cardiac surgery; plasma replacement in exchange tranfusion	Provides immune protection; used to treat patients with low levels of gamma globulin
INCIDENTALS	Does not need to be pooled; 0.9% normal saline may be needed to assist transfusion	Lypholized plasma derivative; obtained by fractionation; allergic reactions reduced over cyro	Also has factors II, VII, X; prepared from large pools of donor plasma; contains Vit-K dependent coagulation factors for treating coumarin overdose in certain patients	5% solution equivalent to plasma; 25% is 5 times the protein concentration of plasma	—	INCIDENTALS Concentrated solution of gamma globulin; prepared from pools of random donors; prepared from donors with large amounts of antibody; extracted from patients exposed to certain viral and bacterial diseases

COMPONENT THERAPY / QUESTIONS

1. Explain how whole blood is used in component therapy.

2. True or false. Whole blood is used to treat a wide variety of diseases and conditions.

3. Briefly discuss the medical meaning of apheresis, citing two kinds of apheresis.

4. Match one component with the condition or conditions it treats.

    a. packed red cells   _____ HLA sensitization
    b. white blood cells _____ blood loss in surgery
    c. platelets   _____ clotting factor deficiency
    d. leukocyte poor   _____ DIC
       red blood cell
    e. cryoprecipitate _____ thrombocytopenia
    f. albumin   _____ hemophilia A
    g. FFP   _____ hypergamma-
                           globulinemia
    h. immune serum _____ hypovolemia
       globulin
    i. coagulation factor _____ HND
       concentrates
    j. PPF   _____ anemia
                           _____ burns

5. What is the name of the additive solution added to packed red blood cells, and when and why is it added?

6. Cyro is a concentrated solution of coagulation proteins found in the plasma. How is it produced?

7. Which of the following do not transmit disease in a transfusion and why? PPF, albumin, coagulation factor concentrates

8. Name four plasma components and four conditions that can be treated with plasma components.

18 SYNTHETIC VOLUME EXPANDERS

Synthetic volume expanders are commercially prepared solutions that are used to replace lost blood volume and plasma fluid. They are normal saline, Lactated Ringer's, dextran, and hespan. When added to the vascular space, synthetic volume expanders increase the volume of blood circulating throughout the body. An adequate circulating blood volume is critical for maintaining life. If blood volume is inadequate, many organ systems, especially the heart, brain, and kidneys, do not function properly.

saline
Lactated Ringer's
dextran
hespan

blood volume

Crystalloids

There are two types of volume expanders: crystalloids and colloids. Each is used differently to treat blood loss. Both are administered IV. The crystalloids (normal saline, Lactated Ringer's, dextrose, and various combinations of these) often are used to replace blood loss, provide fluid for dehydrated patients, and provide direct access to the vascular system for emergency drug administration. Normal saline and Lactated Ringer's are simple solutions made up of anions (negative ions, e.g., Cl^-, HCO_3^- etc.) and cations (positive ions, e.g., Na^+, Mg^{++}, Ca^{++}, etc.). Dextrose is a liquid solution of the simple sugar glucose.

Crystalloids expand the vascular space, but only for a short time. They tend to diffuse into the tissue space (interstitial space) or are filtered out by the kidneys. They may be used when rapid volume expansion is required.

Normal Saline

Normal saline is a naturally occurring salt solution found in the body. It is the only solution that should be transfused along with blood or blood components. It often is infused with blood or blood components because it decreases blood viscosity and does not hemolyze red cell membranes.

Lactated Ringer's

Lactated Ringer's, which is often used as a volume expander, is similar to saline, except that it contains calcium (Ca^{++}) and magnesium (Mg^{++}) ions. It must not be infused at the same time as blood because it contains Ca^{++}, which may stimulate clotting.

Dextrose

Dextrose is a simple sugar solution that often is administered IV to patients. It is never used in blood transfusion because it causes RBCs to hemolyze.

Colloids

Colloids are volume expanders made up of long-chain polysaccharide (sugar and starch) molecules. Due to their molecular size and chemistry, they tend to stay within the vascular system longer than the crystalloids. Colloids resemble plasma more so than crystalloids and are very useful in maintaining blood volume.

They are used to treat certain patients, including burn patients and patients in shock from bleeding, both of whom are likely to be plasma deficient. The colloids include such manufactured substances as Dextran and hetastarch (also known as hydroxyethyl starch or Hespan).

volume replacement

Crystalloids and colloids may be used interchangeably for treating volume replacement. The medical team determines what fluid to use in a given situation.

SYNTHETIC VOLUME EXPANDERS / QUESTIONS

1. What are the chief uses of synthetic volume expanders?

2. Why is adequate circulating blood volume important to maintaining life?

3. Name two kinds of synthetic volume expanders and why they are used.

4. How are crystalloids used, giving two names as examples.

5. True or false. Crystalloids stay in the vascular space for a long time and cannot be used when rapid volume expansion is required. If the answer is false, write the correct version of the statement.

6. Why is normal saline infused with blood or blood components?

7. True or false. Lactated Ringer's must be infused with blood because it contains calcium, which is necessary to stimulate clotting. If the answer is false, write the correct version of this statement.

8. What is the main difference between crystalloids and colloids?

9. What natural blood component do colloids resemble, and why therefore are they useful in treatment?

ANSWERS TO QUESTIONS

THE CONCEPT OF BLOOD, p. 6

1. Red and white cells and platelets, plasma
2. Arteries, veins, and capillaries are the roadways that carry oxygen in the blood from the lungs to the tissues and waste products away from the tissues.
3. Essential in clotting (coagulation) of blood
4. A viscous fluid that is 90% water and 10% solid matter, the latter of which includes carbohydrates, lipids, salts, vitamins, proteins and enzymes
5. Production of blood cells; in the red marrow of bone
6. Each has a unique life span and function when mature, and each is structurally different from the others.
7. Pluripotential and totipotential
8. One daughter cell remains a stem cell to continue the generative process, the other becomes a blood cell.

THE CIRCULATORY SYSTEM, p. 15

1. The circulatory system is a closed loop system of channels in which blood travels throughout the body providing nutrients and oxygen to body organs and tissues.
2. Vascular system; vascular space
3. Arteries, arterioles, veins, capillaries, venules, and indirectly the lymphatic system
4. When blood is ejected from the heart it enters the aorta from which it travels via arteries and arterioles to the organs/tissues. Once in the organs, blood is in the capillary network. Upon leaving an organ, blood enters the venules and veins, which then return it to the heart via two major veins, the inferior and superior venae cavae.

5. The exchange of gases, hormones, nutrients, and waste products between blood and tissues

6. These substances are picked up by the lymphatic system, which returns them to the circulation.

7. To help maintain the body's fluid environment

8. To maintain an equilibrium and to provide nutrients to cells outside it.

9. Lymph nodes

10. Peripheral and cardiopulmonary

11. Venules, veins, superior and inferior venae cavae

12. Endothelial lining or endothelium

13. Blood low in oxygen and high in carbon dioxide

14. Deoxygenated blood returns from the organs and tissues to the right atrium via the inferior and superior venae cavae. Blood in the RA is pumped to the right ventricle through the triscupid valve. From the RV blood is pumped out through the pulmonary valve to the pulmonary arteries and then to the lungs.

15. Oxygen and carbon dioxide

16. Oxygenated blood returns to the left atrium via the pulmonary veins. Blood is pumped from the LA through the mitral, or bicuspid, valve to the left ventricle. From here, blood is pumped out of the aortic valve to the aorta.

THE IMMUNE SYSTEM, p. 25

1. It protects the body from microorganisms and foreign substances by attacking them and rendering them harmless.

2. White; leukocytes

3. Macrophages, granulocytes, T cells, and B cells

4. Phagocytosis is the process whereby a white cell engulfs foreign matter and digests it through its hydrolytic enzymes.

5. It refers to a foreign invader such as bacteria, virus, etc. and also to the chemical on its surface that the body recognizes as foreign.

6. It produces antibodies.

7. An antibody is a chemical complex produced by specialized B cells/plasma cells in response to specific antigens. An antigen-antibody complex is formed when an antigen is recognized by the body and the corresponding antibody binds with the antigen.

8. Immune response

9. Immunoglobulins

10. A B cell matures to a plasma cell, which produces the antibody.

11. IgM: It is restricted to the vasculature because of its size. It is the first antibody produced upon exposure to an antigen. Its main function is to stimulate the complement system. IgD: Little is known about this immunoglobulin. It is believed to trigger antibody synthesis. IgE: It is the immunoglobulin that is produced in excess in people who have allergies. Its main function is to protect the respiratory tract. IgG: This immunoglobulin is divided into four subclasses. (Its main function is to provide protection against both bacteria and viruses.) IgA: This antibody protects the mucus membranes of the body. Its main function is to bind the antigen and then get rid of it when mucin is shed from the mucus membranes.

12. Gamma globulin

13. True

14. Viruses, once inside the cell, are protected from the effects of antibodies because antibodies cannot enter the cell. (It is within the cell that viruses replicate and do most of their damage.)

15. 1) Humoral and 2) cell-mediated

16. Macrophages and neutrophils engulf the foreign matter and render it harmless.

THE ABO BLOOD TYYPING SYSTEM, p. 32

1. By two antigens on the surface of the red blood cell membrane designated A and B

2. Any foreign matter or organism that enters the body and elicits an immune response

3. 1. O 2. AB 3. A 4. B
4. A chemical that is produced by the plasma cells in response to invasion by foreign matter.
5. Anti-A antibody; anti-B antibody; in plasma
6. They have no antigens on their membranes.
7. 1. Anti-B antibody
    2. Anti-A antibody
    3. Neither antibody
    4. Anti-A anti-B-antibody
8. Only in emergencies
9. When the patient experiences shock and even death due to the incompatibility of donor red cells and recepient plasma
10. False. HDN occurs in the second pregnancy after the mother has developed antibodies to the Rh+ factor of the first fetus.
11. RhoGAM

RED BLOOD CELLS, p. 44

1. Erythrocytes
2. In bone marrow
3. 120 days
4. The transport of oxygen from lungs to tissues and carbon dioxide from tissues
5. Hemoglobin; Hgb
6. Hgb is saturated with oxygen in the lungs, and as the RBCs perfuse tissue capillary beds, Hgb releases oxygen.
7. The heme molecule attached to the A and B chains in Hgb is responsible.
8. Hgb's main function is to transport oxygen from the lungs to the tissues (the oxygen-transport capability).
9. 1) Blood flow to the tissues; 2) Hgb concentration; 3) Affinity of Hgb for oxygen
10. If a patient has a low level of Hgb, the physician orders stored blood to return the Hgb to normal.
11. Red blood cells (which contain O_2- carrying Hgb) are added to the vascular space.
12. By lowering Hgb's affinity for oxygen, 2,3-DPG allows Hgb to release oxygen to the tissues.

13. Because stored blood has very low levels of 2,3-DPG and regains only half the normal level in a 24-hour period, the amount of oxygen released to the patient's tissues will be minimal.

14. Its shape gives it the maximum surface for the transfer of gases into and out of the cell. This shape makes for easier travel throughout the body capillaries.

15. Polycythemia, a high RBC cell count, presents circulatory problems because the blood is so thick that it blocks the microvasculature of the lungs and kidneys. Anemia, a low RBC count, means not enough red cells are in the circulation to carry adequate oxygen to the tissues.

16. Hypoxia

17. The kidneys produce erythropoietin, which activates the stem cells to produce RBCs.

18. The percentage of whole blood occupied by the formed elements

19. Cells of the blood system

20. Because it indicates the red cell concentration, Hct provides an indirect measure of the oxygen-carrying capacity of the blood.

21. The number of formed elements in their blood is within the normal range.

22. False. It is three times the value.

23. To dilute the blood

24. The medical team may remove blood prior to surgery if large blood loss is expected and replace it with IV or crystalloid. This procedure hemodilutes the patient. Another time hemodilution is accomplished is during cardiac surgery when the bypass pump is used.

25. 1) Hemodiluted blood flows easily, so better tissue perfusion takes place.
2) Hemodilution increases capillary perfusion.
3) Hemodiluted blood requires less homologous blood, thus reducing patient exposure to disease transmission.

26. The destruction of the red cell membrane

27. 1) The immune response to the wrong blood type used during a transfusion. 2) Bacterial or viral infection. 3) The use of high suction pressure in autologous blood collection.
28. Hgb is released and becomes plasma-free Hgb, which means that it no longer transports oxygen.

WHITE BLOOD CELLS, p. 52

1. Leukocytes
2. Chemotaxis
3. T cells and B cells
4. Infection
5. Phagocytosis
6. Heparin and histamine
7. Skin, lungs, and airways
8. Basophil
9. If a clot forms, WBCs cannot reach the foreign organisms to destroy them, which means the tissue will die.
10. Monocyte
11. They allow the macrophage to digest foreign material.
12. They recognize antigens on the transplanted tissue as foreign, produce antibodies, and destroy the donor organ.
13. They live in the lymph nodes throughout the body.

PLATELETS, p. 54

1. Thrombocytes
2. True
3. To help prevent blood loss, i.e., to maintain the hemostatic process
4. They go to the site and form a plug to help prevent blood loss.
5. They are removed by the spleen.
6. Hemostasis is the bodily process that maintains blood in the vascular system. When blood is lost platelets and chemicals form a network to prevent blood loss by forming a fibrin clot.

PLASMA, p. 59

1. Plasma is the liquid portion of blood in which the formed elements of blood are suspended.
2. Straw-colored; viscous; comprised of solids such as proteins, electrolytes, hormones, and vitamins that are in continuous communication with body tissues
3. Interstitial fluid
4. True
5. More acidic
6. There are health complications for the patient.
7. Sodium
8. It is a source of energy for the cells of the body.
9. It is a hormone that allows sugar to be utilized by the cells of the body (except the red blood cells). It is a source of energy for the cells of the body.

HEMOSTASIS, p. 65

1. They are hemostatic processes that inhibit blood flow from a ruptured vessel. They occur in sequence.
2. Vascular spasm. It is a rapid constriction of the vessel.
3. All responses, or processes, help form fibrin, which holds the clot together.
4. Clot lysis
5. Due to their thick walls, arteries cannot control their bleeding and must be repaired surgically.
6. Contact, adhesion, spreading, ADP release, and aggregation
7. It is a chemical released by the platelet that stimulates other platelets to aggregate to the site of injury.
8. Prostaglandins
9. a. Thromboxane   b. PGI_2
10. It blocks Thromboxane, which prevents ADP release, which prevents platelet aggregation.
11. Platelet membrane phospholipids and tissue membrane phospholipids are activated when tissue is damaged.

COAGULATION CASCADE, p. 75

1. Fibrin formation; clot
2. Either a platelet or tissue phospholipid
3. Both
4. Fibrin would form throughout the body and coagulation factors would be consumed so there would not be enough available for coagulation.
5. The presence of coagulation proteins in the blood available for coagulation
6. It is essential for clotting and provides a bridge for phospholipids to bind proteins.
7. True
8. Intrinsic; extrinsic
9. A series of events
10. Intrinsic: blood removal and contact with a foreign surface (i.e., graft, artificial heart valve). Extrinsic: damaged tissue, cut vessel
11. True
12. It is essential to coagulation and permits coagulation factors to bind calcium. If there is a deficiency, coagulation does not occur.
13. It is an anticoagulant used in the treatment of blood clots.
14. After a vessel has healed the clot must be dissolved by the process of clot lysis so that normal blood flow can return to the vessel.
15. Intrinsic; extrinsic
16. Tissue plasminogen activators
17. When there is rapid bleeding, clots appear, indicating that blood has not had time to react with TPA. When blood loss is slow, blood reacts with TPA and no clots appear.
18. By the circulatory system via cells formed in the liver known as the reticulo-endothelial system.
19. They would act as severe or potent inhibitors of coagulation.
20. They remove FSP from circulation so FSP will not inhibit coagulation.

COAGULATION SYSTEM DISORDERS, p. 81

1. False. They all do.
2. The normal state of vessels that allows blood to flow through uninterrupted
3. In damage to a vessel, surgical or otherwise
4. 1) Trauma 2) Abnormal vessels that interfere with blood flow
5. Hemostasis refers to the prevention of blood loss through processes that inhibit blood flow from a ruptured vessel. Platelets are used in plug formation and also for providing platelet membrane phospholipids.
6. Because fibrin stabilization of the platelet plug does not occur
7. Congenital: single protein abnormality, lasts a lifetime, is hereditary, and is rare. Acquired: multiple factors involved, non-hereditary, and is common
8. Large amounts of tissue phospholipids are released and platelet aggregation is activated. The coagulation cascade consumes platelets and factors. Both clotting and lysis occur.
9. Burns, crush injuries, vasculitis, septicemia, red cell hemolysis
10. Large amounts of coagulation factors are consumed because platelets release phospholipids.
11. When the factors are used up by the body in widespread clotting
12. Clot lysis
13. They become dysfunctional.

PLATELET DISORDERS, p. 84

1. a) If there are not enough platelets, no plug forms over the damaged area and bleeding occurs.
   b) Bleeding occurs if platelet quality is poor, i.e., platelet function is poor.
2. Bone tumors, radiation or chemotherapy, and the immune response to platelets by antibodies against platelets

3. Platelets are used up by the body faster than they can be replaced.

4. Drugs: aspirin, protamine, dextran; Conditions: liver disease, storage damage, FSP

BLOOD TRANSFUSION, p. 94

1. Blood transfusion is the infusion of blood or blood components into patients for the treatment of various surgical and medical conditions. It may be required in the following situations: blood loss during surgery or trauma, hemophilia, internal bleeding, anemia, replacement of a specific component destroyed by chemotherapy.

2. Homologous: someone else's, a donor's; Autologous: one's own

3. Pregnant women, anemics, those with malaria, hepatitis, AIDS, heart disease

4. At least 11-16 g/dl

5. CPD and CPDA-1 are put in blood bags to provide nutrients to RBCs to maintain viability and prevent clotting. Both are referred to as citrate anticoagulant/preservative.

6. Citrate is the anticoagulant that prevents clotting by binding the CA^{++} dissolved in the plasma.

7. CPD — citrate, phosphate, dextrose; CPDA-1 — citrate, phosphate, dextrose, adenine

8. Adenine helps maintain high levels of ATP, a high energy compound that enables the RBCs to provide better O_2 delivery to the tissues.

9. CPD — 21 days; CPDA-1 — 35 days

10. After most of the plasma has been removed

11. False. It can be added only to packed RBCs.

12. 100 mls

13. A+, B-, AB+

14. There is a decrease in the levels of clotting factors, and components become less viable, a condition called storage lesion.

15. The right blood must be administered to the right patient. Blood typing determines blood types; cross matching determines blood type

compatibility between donor and recipient.

16. Compatibility
17. True
18. Hemolyzed red cells, cell fragments, plastic debris, blood clots
19. Leukocyte depletion filter. Some patients, usually those who have received multiple transfusion, react to the Human Leukocyte Antigen (HLA) on the WBC membrane.
20. It reduces blood viscosity and unlike other IV solutions does not hemolyze blood cells.

TRANSFUSION REACTIONS, p. 102

1. Blood donor and recipient types are incompatible; antigens on the red blood cell membrane of the donor react to the antibodies in the recipient's plasma and hemolyze.
2. False. O has no antigens on its red cell membrane.
3. Hemoglobin (Hgb), which is released into the plasma and becomes plasma-free Hgb
4. Flushing, hyperventilation, tachycardia, sense of fright, urticaria, dyspnea, chest pressure, back pain, nausea, vomiting, cyanosis, fever, etc.
5. An incompatible ABO blood transfusion can cause renal shutdown in which the kidneys no longer cleanse the blood and the patient is slowly poisoned.
6. Stop the transfusion immediately.

TRANSFUSION AND DISEASE TRANSMISSION, p. 106

1. Donated blood can contain transmittable bacterial and viral diseases.
2. Hepatitis B and C, syphilis, HTLV-I, HIV
3. False. ELISA measure the antibodies produced in response to the HIV infection and not the virus. A donor may test negative and still carry the virus.

4. False. It is one of several diseases that can be transmitted.
5. The virus inserts the newly formed DNA into the DNA of the host cell, replicates itself, and causes the host cell to produce viruses.
6. Retrovirus
7. He or she has a compromised immune system that allows infections and tumors to appear. Examples include Karposi's sarcoma, *Pneumocystis carinii* pneumonia, thrush.
8. When the opportunistic infections appear, he or she has AIDS.
9. The AIDS virus destroys the T-4 lymphocytes and macrophages, which direct the production of antibodies in the immune system. Without them, the body cannot fight off any disease.

METHODS OF AUTOLOGOUS BLOOD RECOVERY, p. 110

1. Autologous is one's own and does not transmit diseases or cause a transfusion reaction.
2. Predonation, intraoperative blood salvage, and postoperative (wound drainage) collection
3. Cardiac, vascular, liver, and orthopedic, all of which involve significant blood loss
4. False. These are acceptable. Any lower indicate anemia and donation is precluded.
5. It refers to the collection and reinfusion of blood shed by the patient during surgery.
6. Wash and nonwash devices. Wash devices wash the patient's blood before reinfusing it, whereas nonwash devices do not.
7. Heparin, drugs, plasma-free Hgb, hemolyzed red cell membranes, solutions used in surgery, surgical debris
8. Clotting factors, platelets, plasma, and WBCs are washed away and RBCs reinfused.
9. True
10. Blood shed postoperatively can be collected and reinfused, rather than discarded.

COMPONENT THERAPY, p. 122

1. Whole blood is processed into its components (RBCs, WBCs, platelets, and plasma), which are used to treat patients with certain diseases and conditions such as anemia, leukemia, thrombocytopenia, and hemophilia.

2. False. Whole blood is rarely administered to a patient and is done only when blood loss is significant.

3. Apheresis is the removal, or separation, of a specific blood component or components from the circulation for the treatment of a disease or medical condition. A problematic component can be removed and replaced — or not replaced — with an equivalent donor component. Removal of RBCs and WBCs is cytapheresis, or hemapheresis; plasma removal is plasmapheresis; and platelet removal, plateletpheresis.

4. HLA sensitization: d
   blood loss in surgery: a
   clotting factor deficiency: e, g, i, j
   DIC: c, e, g, i
   thrombocytopenia: c
   hemophilia A: e, g, i
   hypergammaglobulinemia: h
   hypovolemia: a, f
   HND: a, f
   anemia: a
   burns: f, g, j

5. After the plasma is removed from a unit of whole blood, ADSOL is added to the packed red cells to keep them metabolically active.

6. During the freezing process of freshly collected plasma, a buffy coat forms on the top. To collect cryo, a unit of FFP is thawed and the precipitate removed.

7. None do; all are pasteurized

8. Components: cryoprecipitate, FFP, coagulation factor concentrates, albumin, PPF, and immune serum globulin; Conditions: liver disease, burns, shock, massive blood loss, bleeding diseases

139

SYNTHETIC VOLUME EXPANDERS, p. 125

1. To replace lost blood volume and plasma fluid
2. Adequate blood volume is necessary for the proper functioning of the brain, heart, kidneys, and other organ systems.
3. Crystalloids and colloids are used to treat blood loss.
4. Lactated Ringer's, normal saline, dextrose, and various combinations of these, replace blood loss, fluid for dehydrated patients, and access to the vascular system in emergency drug administration.
5. False. Crystalloids expand the vascular space but do not stay there long and are used when rapid volume expansion is required.
6. It decreases blood viscosity and does not hemolyze cell membranes the way other crystalloids do.
7. False. Lactated Ringer's should not be infused at the same time because it contains calcium, which may stimulate clotting.
8. Crystalloids do not stay in the vascular space very long; colloids stay longer.
9. They resemble plasma and are very useful in maintaining blood volume.

GLOSSARY

A Blood Type One of four blood groups in humans based on the presence of an antigen on the surface of the red cell. A antigen is on the surface. The plasma of Type A blood contains anti-B-antibody. Type A blood can only receive Type A or O blood.

AB Blood Type One of four blood groups found in humans. It is the least common type found in the U.S. population. Its red cells contain the A and B antigens on their surface. The plasma of AB individuals has no antibodies. Once referred to as the universal recipient, because the individual could receive any blood type.

ABO Blood Group System The most important of several systems for classifying human blood used in blood transfusion therapy.

Acid-Base Balance Refers to the normal equilibrium between acids and bases in the body. It is maintained by buffer systems in the blood plasma and the regulating activities of the lungs and kidneys in excreting wastes, which prevents the build-up of excessive acids or bases in the blood and tissues. With a normal acid-base balance the blood is slightly alkaline or basic.

Active Immunity A form of immunity in which the body provides its own antibodies against disease-causing antigens. It can occur naturally after an infection or artifically after vaccination.

Acquired Immune Deficiency Syndrome (AIDS) A serious, fatal condition in which the immune system is broken down by the HIV virus and does not respond normally to infections. AIDS sufferers often develop Karposi's sarcoma and recurrent severe opportunistic infections such as *Pneumocystis carinii* pneumonia and fungal infections. It is the opportunistic infections that usually kill the victims.

Additive Solutions (ADSOL) Chemicals (dextrose, mannitol, saline, and adenine) added to packed red blood cells. They extend storage life to 42 days. No anticoagulative properties are associated with them. Added only to packed red blood cells.

Adenosine A chemical compound that is a major building block of many biologically active compounds such as DNA, RNA, ADP, and ATP.

Adenosine Triphosphate, or ATP A compound consisting of adenosine, the sugar ribose, and three phosphate molecules. It is involved in many reactions concerning the storage and transfer of energy in cells.

Agglutination The clumping together of antigen-carrying cells or microorganisms as a result of their interaction with antibodies.

Agglutinin An antibody that causes clumping of a specific antigen; for example, the Rh factor in blood.

Alveoli Tiny sac-like structures located in the lung where oxygen and carbon dioxide transfer takes place. They work in very close approximation with the blood capillary network.

Amino Acid An organic compound containing an amino group (NH_2) and a carboxyl group (COOH) that is the basic building block of proteins.

Anaphylactic Shock A severe and sometimes fatal hypersensitivity reaction to the injection or ingestion of a substance to which the organism has become sensitized by previous exposure. Symptoms include weakness, shortness of breath, edema, cardiac and respiratory abnormalities, hypotension and shock. Death may occur within minutes of exposure.

Antibody A complex molecule produced by plasma cells in response to the presence of an antigen. It neutralizes the effect of the foreign matter.

Anticoagulant/Preservative Any solution added to blood to prevent clotting and preserve RBC viability. At present, only CPD and CPDA-1 are available.

Antigen A substance (chemical; protein) or organism that on entering the body causes the production of an antibody that reacts specifically with the antigen to neutralize, destroy, or weaken it

Antigen-Antibody Reaction The process by which the immune system recognizes an antigen and causes the production of antibodies specific to that antigen

Aorta The major artery of the body which leaves the Left Ventricle and delivers oxygenated blood to the tissues of the body

Aortic Valve The three-cusp valve that separates the aorta from the left ventricle

Apheresis The removal of a specific component from a patient for whom it is problematic or for use in medical therapy. Types of apheresis include cytapheresis, plateletpheresis, and plasmapheresis.

Arteriole A small branch of any artery that leads to the capillary network

Autologous Blood Blood that is the patient's own blood. Usually used in reference to the administration of that blood in a transfusion.

Autologous Blood Transfusion The transfusion of one's own blood collected by predonation, intraoperative salvage, or postoperative wound drainage. Eliminates disease transmission and transfusion reactions.

B Blood Type One of four groups of the ABO blood system. It has the B antigen on its surface and the anti-A antibody in the plasma. Can theoretically receive either B or O type blood.

B Cell A lymphocyte important to the production of antibodies in the body when stimulated by an antigen

Bacteria Any of a large group of organisms found in soil, water and air, some of which cause disease in humans and other organisms. Generally classified as rod-shaped (bacillus), spherical (cocci), comma-shaped (vibrio), or spiral (spirochetes).

Basophil A WBC. Normally about 1% of the total white blood cell count, but may increase or decrease in certain diseases

Binding The process whereby two or more chemicals join. The binding of chemicals may activate, inhibit, or neutralize the chemical reaction.

Blood Clot Blood that has gone from the liquid state to the solid state. Clot formation requires integration among many chemicals in the blood — Ca^{++}, phospholipids, and coagulation factors — all of which must be present for a clot to form.

Blood Coagulation The process by which liquid blood is changed into a semi-solid mass, a blood clot. It can occur in an intact vessel, but usually occurs with an injury to a vessel or when blood comes into contact with a foreign surface.

Blood Crossmatching The mixing of the RBCs of a donor with the serum of a potential recipient to determine whether the blood is compatible and can be used for a transfusion. Clumping occurs when incompatible blood types are mixed; it does not occur when that same blood types are mixed.

Blood Transfusion The infusion of blood or blood components into an individual for the treatment of a medical condition, disease, or blood lost due to surgery or trauma. Transfused blood may be homologous or autologous.

Blood Typing A technique for determining a person's blood group. In typing for the commonly used ABO groups, cells and serum are mixed to determine whether or not clumping occurs.

Blood Volume The amount of blood circulating throughout the body in the vascular system. Normal blood volume in the adult is about 5 liters. Maintaining blood volume is essential for organ function of the heart, brain, and kidneys.

Bone Marrow A specialized spongy, fibrous matrix found in the center of bones. Red marrow is involved in the production of blood cells. It is hemopoietic.

Bronchi/Bronchioles The tubes or airways of the lungs that lead from the trachea or windpipe to the alveoli

Capillaries The smallest blood vessels in the body. They connect arterioles and venules. Although only one cell layer thick, the walls of capillaries are used for the transfer of oxygen and nutrients to the tissues and the transfer of waste products and carbon dioxide from the tissues to the capillaries.

Carbon Dioxide A colorless, odorless gas (CO_2) given off by the tissues to the blood, which carries it to the lungs where it is expired. Carbon dioxide levels in the blood regulate the breathing rate and the acid-base balance of the blood. Other body fluids are influenced by the levels of CO_2.

Cell-mediated Response That response brought about by the interaction of a T cell recognizing a foreign invader and stimulating the B cell to produce an antibody

145

Cell Separator The apparatus used in the apheresis process to separate blood components by centrifugating (high speed spinning)

Chemotaxis The movement by a cell or organism toward or away from a chemical stimulus

Clotting Time The time required for blood to clot, usually determined by observing clot formation in a small sample of blood

Coagulation Factor Any of thirteen factors in the blood that is essential for blood to clot. Most coagulation factors are serine proteases and are synthesized in the liver.

Coumadin (Warfarin) A drug used as an anticoagulant in patients who have artificial heart valves or those prone to strokes. It blocks the action of Vitamin K.

Cryoprecipitate The precipitate that is obtained from freezing blood and then thawing it. Cryoprecipitate is the thin white layer that forms at the top of the plasma. It is very rich in factors V, VIII, and fibrinogen.

Cytoplasm The fluid or jelly-like substance found within the cell membrane. The cellular organelles are found suspended in the cytoplasm.

Deoxygenated Blood Blood returning from the body tissues to the heart for circulation through the lungs where it becomes oxygenated

Diapedesis The movement or passage of blood cells through the pores in the intact vessel wall; created by chemical release in response to foreign organisms

Diphosphoglycerate Commonly known as 2,3-DPG, it is a chemical found in the blood bound to the hemoglobin molecule. Functions by allowing Hgb to release oxygen to the tissues more easily.

Disseminated Intravascular Coagulation (DIC) A process that occurs in the body when clot formation and clot lysis happen in a simultaneous uncontrolled fashion. The treatment depends on the cause, but blood products such as platelets, fresh frozen plasma, and cyroprecipitate are used to replace the coagulation factors that are being consumed.

Donation Donating blood for one's own use or someone else's in the treatment of medical diseases and conditions

Electrolyte An element or compound that when dissolved in a solution such as plasma produces ions. Electrolytes are essential for normal physiological processes. NaCl, when placed in solution, separates into Na^+ ions and Cl^- ions.

Endothelium A layer of flat cells that lines blood vessels, the heart, and lymph vessels of the body. A tear or rupture of this layer will stimulate the coagulation system to form a clot.

Enzyme-Linked Immunoassay An initial screening test to determine whether or not blood has antibodies to HIV. If results are positive, further tests (such as the Western Blot) are done to substantiate ELISA.

Eosinophil A type of WBC, normally making up about 1-3% of the total white cell count. Are believed to be abundant in people with allergies.

Erythrocyte A mature RBC that contains the molecule hemoglobin. The main function of the RBC is to transport O_2 and CO_2 between the lungs and the tissues.

Erythropoiesis The process of red cell production controlled by the hormone erythropoietin. This process takes place in the red marrow of bone.

Erythropoietin A hormone produced by certain cells of the kidneys in response to the reduction in the amount of O_2 reaching the tissues. It increases the amount of red cells produced.

Extravascular That area outside the vascular system. Often referred to when speaking about fluid that has left the circulatory system and is in the interstitial space.

Fibrin An insoluble protein in the blood that along with platelets forms a clot. Fibrin is formed by the action of thrombin and its precursor fibrinogen.

Fibrinogen A protein present in the plasma that is essential to the process of blood coagulation. Factor I is converted into fibrin by thrombin in the presence of calcium ions during the process of blood coagulation.

Fibrinolysis The process by which fibrin is broken down into smaller pieces called fibrin split products (FSP) with dissolution of the clot. This is a normal on-going process in the body.

Fresh Frozen Plasma The liquid portion of blood that is removed and frozen immediately. It is used in the treatment of bleeding disorders such as DIC.

Gamma Globulin The most common — and most powerful— antibody (immunoglobulin, IgG); found in the plasma. Provides the chief defense against bacteria, viruses, and toxins. Extracted from donor plasma and commercially processed, it is used for passive immunization.

Globin A protein found in the hemoglobin molecule

Globulin Any of a group of simple proteins found in the blood

Granulocyte A type of WBC, of which there are three types. They are characterized by the presence of granules in their cytoplasm.

H⁺ The ion produced when an acid substance is placed in solutions such as water or plasma. The H^+ must be picked up by a basic solution such as HCO_3^- in plasma.

Hematocrit The measure of the percentage of RBCs as compared with the total blood volume

Hematology The study of blood and blood-forming tissues

Hematopoiesis The process by which blood cells are produced in the marrow

Hemodilution The decrease in the amount of blood in a patient prior to certain surgical procedures. The amount of blood withdrawn is replaced with an equal volume of crystalloid or IV solution.

Hemoglobin (Hgb) A complex protein found in the red cells. It contains the iron pigment heme and the protein globin. It functions by transporting O_2 and CO_2. In the high oxygen content of the lung, O_2 binds with Hgb to form oxyhemoglobin. After depositing O_2 in the tissues and combining with CO_2, it then forms carboxyhemoglobin.

Hemolysis The breakdown of the red cell membrane and the release of Hgb to the plasma. It occurs normally at the end of the red cell's life cycle. It occurs abnormally in certain antigen-antibody reactions, exposure to certain bacteria, in hemodialysis, and in other conditions.

Hemophilia An inherited disease order characterized by excessive bleeding. It occurs almost always in males. There are several forms of the disease: A, B, and C. In all the forms one of the coagulation factors is missing or produced at a reduced rate.

Hemostasis The cessation of bleeding, naturally through coagulation, mechanically with surgical clamps, or chemically with drugs

Heparin A drug used as an anticoagulant for blood. It reacts with antithrombin 3 to produce anticoagulation. It has no anticoagulant effect on its own. It is produced from beef lung or pork mucosa for commercial preparation.

Hepatitis A disease affecting the liver and caused by a virus. It is transmitted through contaminated blood or blood products. It has a mortality rate of 6 - 20%. The virus may remain in the blood for many years, making people carriers and unable to be blood donors. Can cause serious damage to the liver.

Histamine A chemical found in all cells and released in allergic reactions and inflammatory responses. It causes vessels to dilate and decreases blood pressure.

Homologous Blood The blood of another individual, usually in reference to a blood transfusion. Also known as bank blood.

Human Immunodeficiency Virus (HIV) This virus is responsible for the fatal disease AIDS. It belongs to a class of viruses called retroviruses. This group of viruses has RNA as its genetic material; human cells have DNA. The virus contains reverse transcriptase (enzyme) that allows the virus to convert RNA to DNA and insert it into the host cell. HIV mainly attacks the T - 4, or helper lymphocytes, and macrophages, thereby destroying major contributors to the human immune system.

Human Leukocyte Antigen (HLA) An antigen on the WBC membrane that can present problems for patients who have received multiple transfusions. Patients become sensitized to HLA and can experience fever and chills.

Humoral Immune Response The response in the body that causes the production of antibodies

Hydrostatic Pressure The pressure in the capillaries that is determined by the blood pressure, which in turn is directly related to the pressure generated by the heart as it pumps blood.

Hypervolemia An increase in the volume of circulating fluid in the vascular system

Hypothermia The condition in which the body temperature is below 35 degrees centigrade or 95 degrees farenheit. Occurs most often in the elderly and young children when exposed to cold. Hypothermia may be used in some types of surgery to reduce the metabolic requirements of the body and lower oxygen demand.

Hypovolemia A decrease in the volume of fluid circulating in the vascular system. When this situation occurs the patient should be treated with the appropriate fluids, whether blood or cystalloids.

Hypoxia A condition in the body in which there is a decreased amount of oxygen in the tissues. If this continues for any length of time 1) erythropoietin is released from the kidneys, and 2) red blood cell production takes place, thereby increasing the Hgb, which delivers more oxygen to the tissues.

Immune System The system of the body that protects humans from invasion by foreign organisms. It produces antibodies in response to antigens.

Immunoglobulins Chemically complex protein molecules that are also known as antibodies. There are 5 classes, and they are released in a specific sequence.

Inferior Vena Cava The major vein of the body. It receives venous blood from the lower portion of the body and returns it to the right atrium of the heart.

151

Interstitial Space The space in the tissues of the body that separates the cells of the body from one another

Intravascular The term used to describe anything that is located within the circulatory system

Leukocyte The class of blood cells known as WBC, of which there are 5 types. All classes function in conjunction with the immune system to provide defense to the body.

Leukocyte Poor Red Blood Cells Unit(s) of RBCs with WBCs removed to avoid possible sensitization to HLA. There are several ways WBCs can be removed from blood.

Lymphatic System A network of capillary-like vessels, ducts, nodes, and organs that help maintain the fluid environment of the body. The lymphatic vessels have two large vessels, the thoracic duct and right lymphatic duct, that empty into veins in the upper chest and return fluid to the vascular system.

Lymph Node Tissue that acts as a filtering station along the lymphatic channels of the body. These are found throughout the body and are most obvious in the armpits and groin.

Lymphocyte A WBC that normally makes up about 25% of the total white cell count, but increases in the presence of infection. There are two groups of lymphocytes: T cells and B cells.

Macrophage A large WBC that phagocytizes and digests foreign matter and debris that enter the body. It exposes digested antigens on its cell membrane and presents them to the T - 4 cell, which directs antibody production. Some macrophages are fixed in organs such as the liver, spleen, and tissues, while others circulate in the blood.

Megakaryocyte A giant cell found in the bone marrow from which platelets originate by fragmentation of the cytoplasm of the megakaryocyte

Monocyte A WBC that leaves the circulation and enters the tissue. Upon entering the tissue this cell matures into a macrophage.

Mucus A viscous fluid secreted by mucus membranes. It acts as a protective barrier over these membranes, a lubricant that consists chiefly of glycoproteins, particularly mucin.

Nucleus A protoplasmic body in a living cell containing the hereditary material of the cell and controlling the metabolism, growth, and reproduction of the cell. Enucleated: having no nucleus.

Neutrophil A granular WBC that is phagocytic and engulfs bacteria, viruses, and debris. An increase in their numbers occurs during an acute infection.

Nonwash Device Autologous blood recovery system that collects whole blood shed during surgery. When the system is full, blood is reinfused to the patient through a blood filter. No cleansing of the blood occurs.

O Blood Type One of the four types of blood found in the ABO system. It has no antigens on its surface and was once considered the universal donor.

Opportunistic Infection Any infection that attacks an individual with a compromised immune system, as in the disease AIDS

Osmotic Pressure The pressure in the capillary bed (microvasculature) exerted by proteins in the plasma pulling water back into the vascular system. If this phenomenon does not occur, the fluid forced out of the capillaries is not reabsorbed by the vascular system.

Oxygen (O$_2$) A colorless, odorless gas that is essential to all cells of the body for normal respiration and metabolism

Oxygenated Blood Blood that has passed through the lungs and exchanged its carbon dioxide for oxygen. It is pumped from the left ventricle to the various organs and tissues of the body.

Packed Red Cells Blood component derived from whole blood by removing most of the plasma. Now the most common form of blood used in transfusion to replace lost blood or improve anemic conditions. The only component that can be stored in ADSOL.

Parasite An organism that lives on or in the host, deriving nourishment from it. Some cause inflammation, but others cause infection and destroy tissue. Human parasites include fungi, yeast, bacteria, protozoa, worms, and viruses.

Passive Immunity Immunity that occurs when antibodies are produced from sources outside, such as transferring cells or serum from an immunized individual to one who is not immunized. Provided to young children to prevent the development of certain diseases, measles, for example.

Perfuse/Perfusion The passage of fluid through a tissue. Used in reference to blood flow through the lungs where oxygen and carbon dioxide are exchanged.

pH The logarithmic term used to describe the acidity or alkalinity of a solution. It directly measures the H$^+$ concentration of a solution. If the pH is low the solution is acidic; if high the solution is alkaline.

Phagocyte A white blood cell that surrounds and engulfs foreign organisms and debris

Phagocytosis The process by which certain cells engulf and digest organisms. Usually performed by WBCs in response to foreign invaders.

Phospholipids Any of a class of compounds containing a nitrogenous base, phosphoric acid, and a fatty acid. They are found in many cells of the body and function in many important biological reactions, particularly coagulation.

Plasma An acellular, colorless, fluid that is the liquid portion of blood. It consists of water, electrolytes, glucose, fats, and proteins. The formed elements of blood are suspended in this medium.

Plasma Cell A transformed B cell, which is actually the cell that produces antibodies in response to antigen

Plasma-Free Hemoglobin Hemoglobin released from damaged red blood cells. It is released into the plasma where it is removed from the body by the kidneys. May tinge the urine a pink color.

Plasmin The enzyme found in the blood that digests fibrin resulting in clot lysis (dissolution)

Plasminogen The inactive form of plasmin that circulates in the blood until needed to be cleaved into plasmin. It is activated to plasmin by the action of factor XIIa or by tissue plasminogen activator (TPA).

Platelet A disc-shaped, small, enucleated body found in the blood that is essential for coagulation

Polycythemia A serious life-threatening condition characterized by too many RBCs in the circulation, making blood flow through the capillaries difficult. Patients often undergo therapeutic apheresis for removal of the excess RBCs.

Pooled Platelets Platelets collected from multiple donors and mixed together for use in transfusion. Multiple donors increase the chance of disease transmission and transfusion reaction. Often used after bypass surgery.

Pore Size The size of the opening in a blood filter. Filters have different pore sizes depending on their intended use. Standard blood filters in administration sets have pore sizes of 150-270µ. They filter out larger particles. Microaggregate filters have pore sizes that range from 20-40µ and can filter out very small particles.

Red Marrow The hematopoietic marrow found in the center of bones, especially the ribs, pelvis, sternum, and vertebrae.

Renal Failure Also known as kidney failure, this condition occurs when the kidneys no longer cleanse the blood. There are many causes, one of which is an incompatible transfusion reaction.

Reticulo-endothelial System A unit of the body made up of phagocytic cells: Kupffer's cells of the liver, macrophages, and cells of the spleen and bone marrow. They function in the immune response by fighting infection and ridding the body of cellular debris.

Retrovirus A family of viruses with RNA as its genetic material; most organisms have DNA. HIV is a retrovirus.

Rh Factor An antigen present on the RBC of about 85% of people. Persons having the factor are designated as positive. Blood for transfusions must be classified for Rh as well as ABO type.

Right Lymphatic Duct The lymphatic duct that drains lymphatic fluid from the right side of the body and returns it to the circulatory system.

Septicemia The widespread destruction of tissue due to the presence of bacteria or their toxins in the blood. Can be the cause of DIC.

Serine Proteases A term synonymous with the coagulation factors. Describes the type of chemical that the coagulation factors are. Enzymes that cleave, or split, molecules. In coagulation, the splitting of molecules, which thereby confers activity on them.

Serum Plasma minus fibrinogen. If left to stand a sample of blood forms a clot at the bottom of the tube. The remaining fluid portion is called serum.

Single Donor Apheresis A procedure whereby a specific component is removed from a donor's blood and used to treat a disease or condition in another individual

Stem Cell An immortal cell that is able to produce all the cells within the blood system

Superior Vena Cava The major vein of the body that drains the upper portion of the body and returns the blood to the right atrium of the heart

T-4 Tymphocytes A subset of T cells that directs the immune response to foreign organisms

T Cells Small lymphocytes that mature in the thymus and are the chief agents in the cell-mediated immune response. They stimulate B cells/plasma cells to produce antibodies in response to antigen. HIV attacks and destroys the T-4 cells and B cells and thus the body's ability to develop antibodies against the invading organism.

Thoracic Duct One of the two major trunks of the lymphatic system that drains lymphatic fluid from the left side of the body and returns it to the circulatory system

Thrombin A coagulation factor found in the plasma and formed from prothrombin, calcium, and thromboplastin. It acts to change fibrinogen to fibrin and is necessary for clotting.

Thrombocyte A blood platelet. *See* Platelet.

Thrombocytopenia A condition characterized by a lower than normal platelet count. Results in bleeding and easy bruising. The causes of reduced platelets include the use of drugs, neoplastic diseases, and radiation.

Thromboplastin The name for the phospholipid released from damaged tissue and used in the coagulation of blood in the extrinsic pathway of coagulation.

Tissue Plasminogen Activator (TPA) A thrombolytic agent that causes fibrinolysis at the site of clot formation. Currently used to treat acute heart attacks due to blood clot.

Transfusion Reaction The reaction by the body to the infusion of an incorrect blood type. The reaction may be mild or severe, leading to anaphylactic shock and death. The reaction occurs when antigens or blood cells (RBCs, WBCs, and platelets) react with antibodies in the recipient's plasma. The most serious reactions usually involve the RBCs, when transfused cells are hemolyzed.

Vaccine The preparation of a weakened or killed disease-producing virus that is administered by injection or mouth to induce active immunity to a specific disease; for example, the polio vaccine

Vascular Integrity The term used to describe the vessels of the body when they are intact and circulating blood in an uninterrupted fashion

Vascular Space The term used to describe that area occupied by the vessels of the vascular system; used when referring to the blood or fluid in circulation

Vascular System Another name for the circulatory system

Vasculature A term used to describe the vessels of the circulatory system. Most often used in connection with the capillaries, in which case, it is referred to as the microvasculature.

Vasculitis An inflammation in the vessels of the body. Can be caused by a number of situations and can lead to DIC.

Viremia The presence of virus or virus particles in the blood

Virus A small protein-covered core of nucleic acid that is not considered living, but can reproduce itself in the nucleus of the cell. The protein coat is called a capsid.

Vitamin K A fat-soluble vitamin essential for blood coagulation and important in certain energy transfer reactions. It is found in green leafy vegetables, egg yoke, yogurt, and fish liver oils.

Warfarin An anticoagulant with the trade name Coumadin. It is used to prevent and treat blood clots from forming. It works by blocking the action of vitamin K.

Wash Devices The systems used during surgery to collect, wash, and reinfuse autologous blood. They are used in intraoperative blood salvage and in postoperative wound drainage collection. Only RBCs and a small amount of saline are reinfused, all other components are washed into a waste bag.

Whole Blood Blood that has had no components removed from it. It is collected in an anticoagulant/preservative, either CPD or CPDA-1. Usually processed into its components for multiple uses.

Yellow Marrow The non-hematopoietic marrow that is found at the ends of long bones. It consists mainly of fat

APPENDIX

/	= per
g	gram; 454 grams = 1 pound
	28.350 grams = 1 ounce
mg	milligram; 1 milligram = .001 gram
kg	kilogram; 1 kilogram = 1,000 grams;
	2.046 pounds
mM	millimole, or .001 of a mole
	mole = 1 gram molecular weight
	of a substance
liter	1.056 liquid quart
dl	deciliter = .1 liter
ml	milliliter = .001 liter
mm^3	cubic millimeter: 1 mm high, 1 mm long,
	1 mm wide
μ	micron = .000001 meter
mm	millimeter = .25 inch

NORMAL BLOOD VALUES, OR COUNTS

Red Blood Cells

$4.0 - 4.5 \times 10^6/mm^3$ females
$4.5 - 5.5 \times 10^6/mm^3$ males

Hemoglobin

14 - 16 g% females
16 - 18 g% males

Normal Blood Gas Values

	Arterial	Venous
pH	7.35 - 7.45	7.32 - 7.42
pCO_2	35 - 45 mm Hg	41 - 51 mm Hg
pO_2	80 - 100 mm Hg	25 - 40 mm Hg

The term mm Hg means millimeters of mercury pressure. It is the pressure exerted by blood gases in the vascular system.

Plasma-Free Hemoglobin
less than 10 mg/dl

Hematocrit
40 - 44%   females
44 - 47%   males

Total Blood Volume
70 ml/kg adults
90 ml/kg children

White Blood Cells
5,000 - 10,000/mm³
  Neutrophils 60% of WBC count
  Eosinophils 3% of WBC count
  Basophils   1% of WBC count
  Lymphocytes 30% of WBC count
  Monocytes   6% of WBC count

Platelets
150,000 - 400,000/mm³

Electrolytes
  Sodium   138 - 148 mM/L
  Potassium 3.5 - 5.2 mM/L
  Calcium   8.5 - 10.5 mM/L
  Chlorine 98 - 111 mM/L

Glucose
72 - 137 mg/dl

BLOOD CLOTTING TIMES

Partial Thromboplastin Time PTT 24 - 37 seconds
Prothrombin Time PT 10 - 12 seconds
Bleeding Time 9 - 12 minutes
Fibrinogen Level 150 - 350 mg%
Thrombin Time TT +/- 5 seconds of control

BLOOD TESTS TO EVALUATE COAGULATION

Partial Thromboplastin Time

This test measures the intrinsic (long) pathway of coagulation. (A way to remember the pathway this test measures is to think of it as the long pathway and its test as having a long name.) For this test a sample of blood is removed from the patient and placed in a test tube to which platelet factor 3 has been added. The tube is gently heated and then agitated. After the reactants are mixed the timer is started. It is stopped when a fibrin clot appears. If a clot does not appear or clotting time is longer than it should be, an abnormality in the intrinsic pathway is indicated.

Prothrombin Time

This test measures the extrinsic (short) pathway of coagulation. (The name of the test is shorter than that of the test for the intrinsic pathway.) A sample of blood is removed from the patient and placed in a test tube to which tissue thromboplastin has been added. (Tissue thromboplastin stimulates the extrinsic system.) The tube is heated and agitated. After the reactants are mixed, the timer is started. It is stopped when a fibrin clot appears. If a clot does not appear or clotting time is longer than it should be, an abnormality in the extrinsic pathway is indicated.

Thrombin Time

This test measures the final common pathway. It is used to determine the amount or the quality of fibrinogen in the patient's system. A sample of blood is removed from the patient and added to the test tube to which thrombin has been added. The tube is heated and then agitated. The timer is started right after the reactants are added and is stopped when a clot appears. If a clot does not appear or the clot-forming time is longer than it should be, there is an inadequate amount of fibrinogen or there are fibrin split products in the sample.

Fibrinogen Determination
A sample of blood is removed from the patient and added to a test tube to which an abundance of thrombin has been added. The more fibrinogen in the sample, the shorter the time before a fibrin clot appears. If the fibrinogen concentration is low or of an abnormal type, the clotting time takes longer than normal.

Bleeding Time and Platelet Count
The platelet count is performed by looking at a blood smear under a microscope. The number of platelets in the field of view are counted and tells the lab technician the number of platelets in the circulation.

The bleeding time test is performed right on the patient. A blood pressure cuff is placed on the upper arm and inflated to 40 mm Hg of pressure. At the same time, a scratch is made on the underside of the forearm and a timer is started. The blood is blotted away every 30 seconds until bleeding has stopped. When no more blood appears the timer is stopped. Normal bleeding time occurs within 9 - 12 minutes from the beginning of the test. The bleeding time is abnormal if there is an insufficient number of platelets or the quality of platelets is poor.

BIBLIOGRAPHY

Alberts, Bruce, *et al. Molecular Biology of the Cell.* New York and London: Garland Publishing, 1983.

American Medical Association, *Drug Evaluations Annual 1991.* Milwaukee, 1990.

Brown, Barbara. *Hematology Principles and Procedures,* 4th edition. Philadelphia: Lea and Febiger, 1984.

Colby, Diane S., PhD. *Biochemistry: A Synopsis.* Los Altos: Lange Medical Publications, 1985.

Dwyer, John, MD, PhD. *The Body at War.* New York: New American Library, 1988.

Fischbach, D. P., MD, and Fogdall, R. P., MD. *Coagulation, the Essentials.* Baltimore: Williams and Wilkins, 1981.

Ganong, William F. MD. *Review of Medical Physiology,* 9th ed. Los Altos: Lange Medical Publications, 1979.

Hackett, Earle, MD. *Blood.* New York: Saturday Review Press, 1973.

Jandl, James, MD. *Blood : The Textbook of Hematology.* Boston, Toronto: Little Brown and Co., 1987.

Martin Jr., David W., MD; Mayes, Peter A., PhD, DSc; Rodwell, Victor W., PhD; Granner, Daryl K., MD. Los Altos: *Harper's Review of Biochemistry,* 20th ed. Lange Medical Publications, 1985.

Pisciotto, Patricia, MD, Ed. *Blood Transfusion Therapy,* 3rd edition. Arlington, VA: American Association of Blood Banks, 1989.

McMurray, W.C., PhD. *A Synopsis of Human Biochemistry With Medical Applications.* Philadelphia: Harper and Row, 1982.

Ream, Allen, MD, and Fogdall, R., MD. *Acute Cardiovascular Management.* Philadelphia: J. B. Lippincott and Co., 1982.

Reed, C. and Clark, D. *Cardiopulmonary Perfusion.* Houston: Texas Medical Press, 1975.

Rossi, Ennio C., MD; Simon, Toby L., MD; Moss, Gerald S., MD., eds. *Principles of Transfusion Medicine.* Baltimore: Williams and Wilkins, 1991.

Sage, David, MD. *Anaphylactoid Reactions in Anesthesia.* Vol 23, No 3. Boston: Little Brown and Co., 1985.

Scott, Andrew. *Pirates of the Cell.* New York: Basil Blackwell, Inc., 1987.

Shapiro, Barry, MD; Harrison, Ronald, MD; and Walton, John, R.R.T. *Clinical Application of Blood Gases.* Chicago, London: Yearbook Medical Publishers, 1985.

Smith, James, MD, and Kampine, John, MD. *Circulatory Physiology.* 2nd edition. Baltimore: Williams and Wilkins, 1984.

Stryer, Lubert, PhD. *Biochemistry.* San Francisco: W. H. Freeman and Co., 1975.

Valeri, C. Robert, MD. *Physiology of Blood Transfusion.* Boston, MA: Naval Blood Research Laboratory, Boston University School of Medicine, March 1, 1989.

Walker, Richard H., MD, editor-in-chief. *Technical Manual,* 10th Ed., 1990. Arlington, VA: American Association of Blood Banks.

West, John, MD, PhD. ed. *Best and Taylor's, Physiological Basis of Medical Practice.* 11th edition. Baltimore: Williams and Wilkins, 1985.

Williams, William, MD, *et al. Hematology.,* 4th ed. New York: McGraw Hill, 1990.

Wintrobe, Maxwell, MD. *Clinical Hematology.,* 5th ed. Philadelphia: Lea and Febiger, 1961.

INDEX

A blood type, 141
AB blood type, 141
ABO Blood Group System, 141
ABO blood typing, 27-31
    RH factor, 29-31, 142
    for typing, 90
acid-base balance, 141
acidosis, 57
acquired factor deficiencies, 78
Acquired Immune Deficiency Syndrome (AIDS), 141
    enzyme-linked immunoassay (ELISA) blood test, 103
    role of T-4 lymphocytes and macrophages, 105
    and transfusions, 86, 87, 103-105
active immunity, 141
additive solutions, 88-89, 142
adenine, 87, 88
adenosine, 142
adenosine triphosphate (ATP), 88, 142
ADSOL, 88-89, 114, 142
agglutination, 142. See also clumping
agglutinin, 142
agglutinogen, 132
AIDS. See Acquired Immune Deficiency Syndrome (AIDS)
albumin and plasma protein fraction (PPF), 117-118
allergic transfusion reaction, 96
allergies and IgE antibody, 19, 48
alveoli, 13-14, 142
American Blood Bank Association, 89
amino acid, 142
anaphylactic shock, 142
anemia, 39
antibodies, 18-20, 22, 142
  anti-A and anti-B, blood typing, 27-28
    RH factor, 29-31
anticoagulants, 68, 72, 143
  and donated blood, 87-88
antigens, 17-18, 143
    A and B, blood typing, 27-29, 90
    antigen-antibody complex, 18-20
    antigen-antibody reaction, 96, 143
aorta, 7, 8, 12, 143
aortic valve, 143